WHAT'S MISSING IN MEDICINE

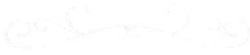

WHAT'S MISSING IN MEDICINE

Unleashing the Healing Power of the Subconscious Mind

C. V. TRAMONT M.D.

DU LAC PUBLISHING, LLC

Copyright © 2016 C. V. Tramont M.D.

Library of Congress Registration Number TXu 1-913-451

ISBN-13: 9780996819527
ISBN-10: 0996819525

This book is dedicated to all the caring and compassionate physicians in the medical profession who maintain an open mind when it comes to understanding and utilizing a diagnostic and therapeutic regime that has shown itself to be safe and extremely successful.

Apathy is not an option.

TABLE OF CONTENTS

The author would like to express his gratitude for these endorsements from caring and compassionate physicians who maintain an open mind in regard to Comprehensive Hypnoregression Therapy:

"I am finding that in today's medicine you have to have more knowledge, experiences and tools in the 'Doctor's Black Medicine Bag' in order to fully understand and treat your patient. The soul of the patient should be addressed and not overlooked. It would be like constructing an elaborate golden temple only to have a dark empty cold interior. All humans have their own story, each head is a world in itself, and everybody wants to know the meaning of their life and of those around them. Dr. Tramont's research, work, and writings address the health of the soul and how it relates to our wellbeing." ---- Gilbert M. Garcia, D.D.S., MPH, M.D. (Pediatrician)

❦

"My name is Dr. Nisim John and I am the founder and Medical Director of Integrative Cancer Therapy Centers as well as Integrative Medical Centers. I have always been an advocate of non-toxic, safe and effective therapies to help, heal and cure people from diseases whether emotional, physical or spiritual. Many years ago I had the blessing and privilege to meet Dr. Charles Tramont, and not only sit in on his treatment sessions but also be part of one myself. The experience was incredible. Going to conventional medical school, I had at that time not been exposed to this type of therapy that helps patients with diseases on all levels. Dr. Tramont's Comprehensive Hypnoregression Therapy is a wonderful and effective modality that I recommend for the helping, the healing and the curing of ill patients. Dr. Tramont's book *What's Missing in Medicine: Unleashing the Healing Power of the Subconscious Mind* should be part of every physician's library." ---- Nisim John, M.D. (Medical Director of Integrative Cancer Therapy Centers and Integrative Medical

Centers, Independent Researcher, International Conference Speaker, Educator, and Consultant)

❧

"By using Comprehensive Hypnoregression Therapy, Dr. Charles Tramont offers his patients an effective alternative therapeutic modality that is real and undeniably efficacious without toxic pharmaceuticals and laborious counseling. Whether a skeptic or not, the reader of his new book will discover a powerful tool that can potentially awaken a sleeping soul and provide answers to many life questions that can bring permanent healing to self and others. His stories are powerful and convincing, his experiences unique and true, and his compassion refreshing and moving." ---- Elliot Shin, M.D., M.S. (Family Physician and Nuclear Physicist)

❧

"As a physician who graduated from Beijing Medical College, earned a PhD in physiology and biophysics from the Medical College of Ohio, and is now practicing medicine in America, I have been exposed to many successful traditional and alternative methods of treating illness. I applaud Dr. Charles Tramont's courage not only to brave new frontiers in hypnotherapy but also to share the stunning results of his research and practice in *What's Missing in Medicine*. By applying his creativity, innate bravery, and his keen listening skills which were honed in his OB/GYN practice, Dr. Tramont developed and utilizes a broader application of hypnosis which he calls Comprehensive Hypnoregression Therapy. He is offering the medical community an innovative and effective modality which has already proved helpful to many individuals known to me." ---- Wen Guo, M.D., PhD. (Internal Medicine)

❧

"Dark negative force removal, i.e., 'Entity/Demonic force removal,' is one of the most difficult and challenging areas for hypnotherapists and not so many practitioners seem to choose to enter in this specialty. After positively identifying the force, one has to effectively remove it with various techniques. The negative force could be sneaky, deceptive, manipulative and extremely powerful. In order to specialize in this area, the practitioners need to have the precise technique, courage, conviction, strength, knowledge, wisdom, commitment and the strong desire to serve humanity. Dr. Tramont has all of them. Looking back at his unique combination of background, he demonstrated his leadership skills as an Air Force colonel, his precision technique as a flight surgeon, and his compassion as an OB/GYN physician. His practice of many years have already helped a lot of people in the whole world. He is genuine. How fortunate we are to have Dr. Tramont here and now!" ---- Grace K., M.D. (Board Certified in Internal Medicine, Holistic Medicine, Medical Acupuncture, and Clinical Hypnotherapy)

"Dr. Tramont explores and delivers an understanding of the human experience that is rarely discussed in Medical Schools around the world. Drawing on decades of experience as an Obstetrician and hypnoregression therapist, Dr. Tramont takes us on a departure from allopathic medicine and its limitations to explore exciting areas of therapy that deal with spirituality, healing and the soul head on. His ideas and therapy may be considered unconventional, but Dr. Tramont is a leader amongst a brave few practitioners who are willing to question the status quo of the house of medicine in order to deliver life changing outcomes to those who are most in need." ---- Elad Bicer, M.D. (Emergency Medicine)

"I'm 48 years of age and my entire life have been surrounded by people that have introduced me to my past life memories. I'm a better person, father, spouse and friend of the world because of it. Finding a practical mechanism that can help my patients that are truly suffering will not only be a great joy, but is also a very large missing piece of western medicine." -- Sean McFadden, M.D. (Obstetrics and Gynecology)

❦

"The time has come for all physicians to recognize the critical role of karma and previous lives as root causes of virtually all significant illnesses. I have often said that, if I had only one therapy to offer, I would choose Past Life Therapy. Perhaps those physicians who still reject this tremendously useful technique need a session with Dr. Tramont to discover the cause of their stubborn refusal to recognize Truth! Everyone needs the benefit of this magnificent spiritual healing approach." ---- C. Norman Shealy, M.D., Ph.D., (Neurosurgeon; President, Holos Energy Medicine Education; Founder and first President of American Holistic Medical Association; inventor of the TENS Unit)

❦

"The knowledge of Medicine is growing exponentially but often treating the "whole" patient is lacking. The alternative approach used by Dr. Tramont has helped many patients to be healed and find well-being. His hypnoregression therapy has aided many patients to be healed without drugs or years of counseling. The cases are fascinating and offer insight into how the subconscious can produce very real physical disease. The work and research that has been done by Dr. Tramont gives insight into the nature of our soul and gives an alternative therapeutic approach that will help many." ---- David Lee Wilson, M.D, (Anesthesiology)

"Dr. Charles Tramont's new book *What's Missing in Medicine* has laid the groundwork for a more holistic view of a person including the soul with the mind and body. His years of past life hypnoregression therapy experience bring new tools to intervene in refractory emotional health problems with many documented cases. In a more general vein, I am very positive about benefits to all souls. Remember, "You don't have a soul. You are a soul. You have a body." C.S. Lewis" ---- Blair Holder, MD (Internal Medicine)

"Being a doctor that specializes both in alternative and Family Medicine made me realize that conventional medicine does not have all the answers to illnesses. We often forget that we should not only treat the body but also the soul and subconscious mind. I have personally witnessed the hypnoregression therapy of Dr. Tramont and I am amazed at how the subconscious mind really affects someone's life and relationships. I can sincerely say that if this can be a part of regular mental therapy then nobody will be taking anti-depressants and anti-anxiety pills and perhaps avoid suicides and homicides. I do believe this can be a great armamentarium for every doctor. Everybody should be reading this incredible book." ---- Divina Gracia Averilla-Obena, M.D., FAAFP, ABAARM

Chapter 1

THE SPIRITUAL EVOLUTION OF A PHYSICIAN

You are about to bear witness to a journey that I have taken on a path I could not say no to. Surely you, along with many others, will have one of several reactions to what I am attempting to accomplish. Because of cultural and academic perspectives, these reactions may include being shocked, being disturbed, or just being relieved that conventional medicine, which has made some advances in becoming holistic, is now hearing from one of its own, that it should be open to a form of diagnosis and treatment that will cure people, save lives, and save money.

What I am saying here is that medicine has come a long way in advancing the health and longevity of man's physical body but has not taken into consideration the fact that man has a soul, which is irrevocably linked to his consciousness. I have come to believe that the soul is the spiritual energy that enables a human being to think, to feel, and to carry out actions, all of which contribute to his personality and to his very life. It is the part of us that lives on in a spiritual dimension following the death of the physical body.

I was a conventional physician specializing in obstetrics and gynecology for over thirty two years. I have seen thousands of patients, delivered thousands of babies, and performed thousands of surgeries, and thus am able to speak from experience about these endeavors. To date I have conducted hypnotic regressions for over twenty three years. I have learned that there is no distinction of time in the spiritual dimension and that the past, the present, and the future are all occurring simultaneously. This is a hard concept for many individuals to grasp, but it certainly explains why a very small percentage of people are also affected by past present-life and future-life memories. I have found that the great majority of painful memories that affect people are past life memories, and I therefore will be referring primarily to past life memories throughout this book.

I find that I have also come to a time in my life when I can now speak from extensive experience in regard to carrying out thousands of what I call *Comprehensive Hypnoregressions* with the patient under deep hypnosis. I have named this form of diagnostic and therapeutic treatment *Comprehensive Hypnoregression Therapy* because it must not only consider past life causes of people's problems, it must also include discovery, identification, and removal of another very important cause: *foreign energy*.

Foreign energy comes from external sources and attaches to people, most of whom are unaware of its presence. Some individuals suspect the presence of something but are unable to identify the source. Foreign energy is composed of human and non-human entities which will draw energy from the person and adversely affect him both physically and emotionally. In the coming chapters we will discuss the various forms of attached foreign energy in detail.

My experience has proven to me that a large percent of human beings are suffering from the negative influence of highly emotional past life memories that have been recalled by the subconscious mind and/or from the detrimental influence generated when one is affected by attached entities. I have witnessed unbelievable sequelae from such past life trauma and entity interference, resulting in emotional, mental, and physical illness. These injurious influences have been stopped and the patient cured of these maladies in a very large percent of patients using such therapy. I firmly believe that medicine must consider this etiology and its treatment seriously. Too many physicians and those in teaching positions remain aloof to the subject of spirituality and continue to fear ridicule by their peers if they dare to discuss such subjects.

I am aware that the controversial material to be presented here will very likely challenge the reader's belief system, as it has challenged mine along the way. I am also aware that I may be subjected to criticism by some of my colleagues; however, this is a critique I am well prepared to defend, mostly because of having witnessed the healing of a massive number of patients who had emotional and physical ailments which conventional medicine was unable to effectively treat. The relief of suffering is why I went into medicine in the first place; and since this process works, I feel called to share what I have learned.

In some cases prescription drugs can be helpful to calm patients so as to enable their minds to undergo a comprehensive hypnoregression session and utilize the subconscious mind to honestly address their issues, face their problems head on, and overcome the obstacles which have prevented them from attaining peace and happiness. Such actions lead to cures.

Healing oneself through the power of the mind is not so far-fetched. It just takes a well-trained person who will use the power of the patient's mind to heal the patient. The therapist accomplishes this miraculously therapeutic feat through the use of Comprehensive Hypnoregression Therapy. You will be impressed with the way in which the conscious mind interfaces and integrates with the subconscious mind so as to allow patients to release whatever is causing their problems. I feel very strongly that the answers to people's difficulties lie within the subconscious mind, which is accessible through deep hypnosis and is capable of identifying the causes of these problems. If the cause is identified as a past life memory that has surfaced, the patient's conscious mind understands why the problem occurred and that it happened a long time ago. The conscious mind is now able to release the effect, thus allowing anxiety to be reduced, the autonomic body systems to function better, and the immune system to improve (or as the new generation might say, the immune system is able to "reboot"). If the cause is an attached entity, it is removed, and the problems leave with it. This treatment modality is a dynamite weapon in the war against physical and emotional illness.

The U. S. Secretary of Health and Human Services adopted certain sets of international codes that were to be used for diagnosis and for procedures. These specific codes include ICD-9 and ICD-10, both of which are part of the International Classification of Diseases (ICD), which is used for epidemiological, clinical, and health management purposes. These ICD codes are also able to monitor many aspects of human disease, including their incidence and prevalence, thus providing statistics on mortality and morbidity for the World Health Organization members.

Use of these International Classification of Disease (ICD) codes is required by the Health Information Portability and Accountability Act (HIPAA) and has to follow a certain international standard of coding for reporting to the World Health Organization, which is the directing and coordinating authority for health in the United Nations system, thus providing leadership on global health. The ICD-10-CM code has been in place in many countries for several years and was fully implemented in the United States effective as of October 1, 2015, officially replacing the ICD-9-CM code. The updated 2016 ICD-10-CM diagnosis code F-44.89 is entitled "Other Dissociative and Conversion Disorders," one of which is a "disorder of trance and possession."[1]

According to Richard Saville-Smith, MA, MSc, a student at the University of Edinburgh in Scotland working towards a doctoral degree, "Possession trance involves replacement of the customary sense of personal identity by a new identity, attributed to the

---

1 http://www.icd10data.com/ICD10CM/Codes/F01-F99/F40-F48/F44-/F44.89; 1/28/2016

influence of a spirit, power, deity, or other person and associated with stereotyped 'involuntary' movements or amnesia and is perhaps the most common Dissociative Disorder in Asia."[2]

People suffering from phobias, anxiety, depression, insomnia, and a host of many other stressful symptoms will often seek treatment because their ability to function normally is impaired in occupational or social settings, or in personal relationships. Diagnostic workups on patients with these problems are often unsatisfactory because of the limitations of conventional medicine. I firmly believe that an examination of the patient's subconscious mind is crucial in these situations and will often reveal the cause to be due to an entity or a past life memory. Using Comprehensive Hypnoregression Therapy in this way would be both diagnostic and therapeutic.

The majority of religious teachings in the world today endorse reincarnation and karma. Most cultures include the concept of spirit possession. The Roman Catholic Church has been conducting exorcisms for hundreds of years and is now calling for more priests to be trained to perform exorcisms. *Possession* is usually defined as being taken over or controlled by an evil spirit, also referred to as a demon or a dark force. Exorcism in the Catholic Church is all about removing evil spirits from a person who is "possessed;" however, the term *possession* is also used, and occasionally defined, as being dominated or at least influenced by spirits, demons, or other supernatural beings. Academic institutions and most people in all walks of life will use the term "possession" in this way. I feel that the preferable description of a spirit, demon, supernatural being, etc., influencing a person would be to refer to it as "entity attachment" and specify the type of attachment; however, the term "possession" appears to have become a synonym for entity attachment and should now be considered as such in present-day usage.

---

2 Saville-Smith, Richard. "Releasing the Spirits - The Implication of Cultural Accommodation," Academia.edu on March 27, 2013. [http://www.academia.edu/3126064/Releasing_the_Spirits_-_The_implications_of_cultural_accommodation]

I – and others who have removed entities from a large percent of people that we have seen – know without reservation that the experience of entity attachment is an extremely common occurrence that adversely affects people, causing them emotional and physical distress, while they remain completely unaware of the presence of these entities. We are also aware that cultures and religions have a minimal influence on whether an entity will attach to an individual. Entity attachment occurs due to the vulnerability of people to such attachments. This will be discussed in the next few chapters. People rarely seek treatment from a physician because they feel that they are possessed; they seek treatment because they have one or more of a vast array of symptoms which are often caused by attached entities. These symptoms often depend on the amount and type of entity attachments present, or as some people would say, the "degree of possession." The greater the degree, the greater the symptoms. Fortunately, people who have an exceptional amount of attached entities are nowhere as common as those with a minimal number of entities present; however, even one or two entity attachments can modify a person's behavior by altering his attitude and emotions. This will often ignite strong negative feelings, including fear or anger, and bring about anxiety, depression, and a host of symptoms that cannot be explained nor helped with medications.

The United States is a young country when compared to cultures throughout the world that have existed for thousands of years; these cultures appear to have a greater understanding of the spirit realm and its influence on human beings. I have seen patients from these cultures who were quite knowledgeable about spirit possession and felt that depossession was needed to resolve their physical and emotional problems.

BASIC DOCTRINES OF OUR SPIRITUAL REALITY

When I wrote my book *From Birth to Rebirth*, I was very passionate about the basic principles of our spiritual reality, namely the doctrines of reincarnation and karma. Many authors have exhausted the seemingly endless succession of ramifications that stem from the belief in reincarnation, namely various perspectives and world views on important topics such as cultural and religious war, abortion, homosexuality, discrimination, and the environment. My experience with these subjects is very much in agreement with these authors; however, since I enjoy being creative in my approach to many situations, my hypnotic regression sessions have become much more comprehensive and occasionally experimental. Thus my personalized approach to this fascinating and therapeutic doctrine of spiritual reality has resulted in extensive experience, which has now become my reality.

Reincarnation can be defined as the rebirth of the soul into a new body. This rebirth is complimented by the presence of the spiritual doctrine of karma, derived from the Sanskrit word *karman*, meaning deed or act. Sanskrit is the ancient Aryan language that originated with the Hindus of India. Karma is the aggregation, the amassing of all of one's deeds that have occurred during all the incarnations of one's existence and the effect of those deeds upon that soul. It has to do with cause and effect. It is the balance of energy that teaches us that we are responsible for what we do, and its effect in determining our fate is profound. In a way, karma is our spiritual inheritance. It weighs actions that are good against those actions that are evil, actions that help others against those that hurt others, and actions that bring harmony to the universe against those that bring disharmony. It is justice in the truest sense. The present reality that we create for ourselves and others will be back in kind in a future time. In my mind karma is not there to punish us, rather it is in place to teach us.

The general thinking is that negative karma that occurred in a previous life will always generate negativity in one's present life. My thoughts on this are that enlightenment brings on wisdom, which in turn creates understanding that can lead to intentions that stem from love and compassion. I believe such intentions can alter the effects of the karmic balance and possibly eliminate them.

When people are aware that they are responsible for their actions and know that they have been given the greatest gift of all, namely free will, they know without reservation that they cannot be victims, and they can only blame themselves for what happens. People must realize that they are creating karma every moment of their life, and it isn't just through actions; it is also through thoughts and intentions, which may or may not lead to actions.

Enlightened individuals usually have a firm belief in reincarnation. Twenty-five years ago I had no opinion about reincarnation except that I thought it was a cool idea, even though my religion labeled it heresy. Since that time I have proven to myself that reincarnation is quite real. This proof came about from validation of countless cases of people's lives in past times through hypnotic regression. I have also witnessed the speaking of languages unknown to the patient.

YOUNG CHILDREN WHO REMEMBER PAST LIVES

A story that I've been hearing about in the news over the past few years involves a young boy by the name of James Leininger. It seems that James had a passion for airplanes ever since he was very young. At 20 months old James had been brought to an airplane exhibit and wanted to keep going back to the section on World War II memorabilia. He even refused to leave after three hours. By the age of two he was playing with toy airplanes exclusively. His parents, Andrea and Bruce Leininger, said that this activity began to give him frequent nightmares, causing him to scream in the middle of the night. One such night his mother woke him up and asked him what he was dreaming about. His response was, "Airplane crash! Plane on fire! Little man can't get out!"[3] A video of him at age three shows him going over a plane as if he were doing a preflight check. James' mother pointed to an area on the underside of a new toy airplane

---

3 Leininger, Bruce and Andrea, with Ken Gross. *Soul Survivor.* Grand Central: NY, NY, 2009, p. 11

and called it a bomb. James immediately corrected her and said that it was a drop tank.

The nightmares worsened and became more frequent, so James' parents took him to see a counselor and therapist. As a result the nightmares lessened, and James became more detailed in his description about his alleged past, mostly before going to sleep. James said that his airplane had been hit by the Japanese, and it crashed. He said that he flew a Corsair and later said that the Corsair used to get flat tires all the time. One night James told his father that the name of the boat he took off from was the Natoma, and Jack Larson was the name of someone he flew with. Later James said that he had been shot down at Iwo Jima, and his plane took a direct hit on the engine.

James' father, Bruce Leininger, did some research and discovered that the Natoma Bay was a small aircraft carrier that was deployed in the Pacific and Jack Larson was one of the pilots that flew off of the Natoma Bay and presently is living in Arkansas. This and other confirmations of the validity of his son's past life blew Bruce Leininger's mind.

Obsessed with the need to find out more, Bruce Leininger researched military records and spoke to men who had served aboard the Natoma Bay. He found out that a James M. Huston, Jr., was the only pilot from the squadron killed at Iwo Jima. James' father then contacted Ralph Clarbour, a rear gunner on an American airplane that also took off from the Natoma Bay, who said his plane flew next to the one flown by James M. Huston, Jr., during a raid near Iwo Jima on March 3, 1945. Clarbour said he saw Huston's plane struck by anti-aircraft fire, and added, "Huston's plane was hit right in the engine."[4]

James continued to come up with knowledge and experiences that were way beyond a child's recollection. James' mother stated that on a day she was preparing meatloaf and told James that this would be the first time for him to eat it, James retorted that he

---

4 Ibid., p. 223

hadn't had meatloaf since he had been on the Natoma. Also, James had three GI Joe dolls that he named Leon, Walter, and Billy. Research revealed military records which recorded the names of three pilots from the Natoma Bay squadron that had previously lost their lives in other battles, Lieutenant Leon Stevens Connor, Ensign Walter John Devlin, and Ensign Billie Rufus Peeler. James was asked why he came up with these names for his GI Joe dolls. His answer was, "Because that's who met me when I got to Heaven."[5]

At this point James' father now says he believes his son was James M. Huston, Jr., in a past lifetime. The Leiningers wrote a letter to Huston's sister, Anne Baron, regarding everything that has transpired, and now she is also a believer. Huston's sister sent James some of James Huston's personal effects that were sent home after the war; namely, a bust of George Washington and a model of a Corsair aircraft. James' parents, Bruce and Andrea Leininger, overcame their original skepticism and have broadened their belief system in regard to reincarnation and as a tribute to this spiritual enlightenment, they with the help of Ken Gross, have written a book about this remarkable story of reincarnation titled *Soul Survivor*.

Before leaving this subject I would like to mention Dr. Ian Stevenson and his well-known collection of scientific data that strongly supports reincarnation. What we are talking about here is forty years of scientific investigation with over three thousand cases of children who consciously and spontaneously recalled past lifetimes. A good number of these children spoke languages that were unknown to them, some of which were ancient languages and there was never any evidence of previous exposure to those languages. These children were from all parts of the world, and at least half of them were from cultures that denied the existence of reincarnation. The late Ian Stevenson, M.D., was a professor and Chairman

---

5 Ibid, p. 157

Emeritus of the Department of Psychiatry at the University of Virginia. He devoted the latter part of his life to this scholarly and most respected endeavor.

DEFINITE EVIDENCE OF PREVIOUS LIFETIMES

A few years after the turn of the century I spoke to a professional hypnotist by the name of Irvin Mordes. He was in his nineties at the time but was extremely sharp and very proud of the fact that he had regressed a subject back to sixteen lifetimes, and the subject was able to speak sixteen different languages and write in all those languages while under hypnosis. Irvin told me that he repeated this session in a research center with several physicians in attendance who were there to witness this regression. The subject was a 32-year-old man who had a tenth grade education and knew only the English language. The case became quite famous and stands as an undeniable proof of reincarnation. A summary of this case follows as a quote from the book *Hypnotherapy Encyclopedia* by Ormand McGill, PhD. It is from the chapter titled *"Evidence of Previous Lifetimes"*:

> The case of Alan Lee, a Caucasian man born in Philadelphia May 4, 1942, provides the best objective evidence of the fact of reincarnation. Alan Lee never completed school beyond the tenth grade and never had learned any other language besides English.
>
> In research conducted at Maryland Psychiatric Research Center, 1974, Alan was regressed to sixteen previous lives by professional hypnotist Irvin Mordes. All of the sessions were witnessed and affirmed by the physicians and researchers who affixed their signatures: Walter Tauke, M.D., Jerome Rubins, M.D., Edward L. Reed, M.D., Ruth Martin, John H. Metzinger, Victor Schlector, M.D., and Walter Panhnke, M.D.

With each previous life regression came an uncanny ability to speak and write in the language of whatever period of history he was re-experiencing. Half of the languages he expressed, which had not been taught for centuries, were checked for accuracy. In the hypnotic state Alan spoke and wrote fluent American English, rural English, ancient English, Italian, Cherokee Indian (Tehalgic), Norman French, idiomatic Latin, classic Greek, Hebrew, Egyptian Hieroglyphics, Egyptian Demotic, Egyptian Hieratic, Atlantean, and Lemurian. He was regressed back each time and requested to write a description of his memory in the manner of the writing of the time. The ancient scripts of his handwriting are persuasive, factual evidence of previous lives.

During this study, Alan's vital signs were carefully monitored. His blood pressure would suddenly drop from his normal 120 over 80 to 60 over 30 and his pulse decreased. Such a reaction may be normally associated with a state of shock, but no such thing occurred. He was fine in every way.[6]

I have always said that we will never know how the spirit world works until we're there, but I am convinced that reincarnation is an important part of our soul's destiny. The following paragraphs represent a simplification of my beliefs in regard to reincarnation and how I have been made to understand how it works, according to my experience with patients.

Our Creator, who is absolute perfection and the consciousness of all that is, creates many souls in order to manifest. All of these eternal souls have a spark of the Creator within them but are no longer perfect, since they are now separated from the Creator. Each individual soul is pure energy, and as such, vibrates as all energy does;

---

6 Ormond McGill. *Hypnotherapy Encyclopedia*. Palos Verdes, CA: Creativity Unlimited, 2001. p. 633

however, each soul maintains its own specific vibration, and this vibrational frequency will increase as the soul attains perfection so it may once again be with the Creator, its ultimate goal. Perfection can be accomplished when the soul has mastered the learning of many lessons such as love, compassion, forgiveness, patience, and so on. The soul may choose to learn these lessons in the afterlife, which has often been described as a school of sorts, or it may choose to learn these lessons by incarnating as a living being on any planet in the universe, including Earth.

A council of Master Spirits is often called together to help an individual soul choose its lesson or lessons. Master Spirits are very advanced in perfection and no longer have to incarnate; they devote themselves to helping other souls. The soul has been given the gift of free will, enabling it to make choices about everything. If the soul chooses to incarnate on Earth it will then take part in a planning stage where it will make choices regarding every aspect of the life to come, including parents, gender, location, intelligence, race, health, and ultimately every aspect of its physical being, all for the purpose of learning lessons. Eventually the soul joins with its physical body in the mother's womb.

My experience with patients has given me the definite impression that life on Earth is not easy; however, when lessons are learned during a life on Earth, they are learned well. Many souls fail to learn these lessons and have to return to another lifetime on Earth to accomplish this. Occasionally a soul may continue to return to Earth many times over in order to learn the same lesson. Eventually the soul will 'get it right' and then work on other lessons.

Agreements may be made with other souls in the same soul group (a soul group is a gathering of souls who have made agreements to incarnate with each other in certain lifetimes, usually for the purpose of resolving karmic issues). When this occurs, and these souls cross paths in a lifetime, people experience an indescribable feeling of being connected and drawn to each other; however, many individuals ignore these feelings and allow these rare opportunities to pass them by.

MY OBJECTIVE

My goal in writing this book is to show how valuable Comprehensive Hypnoregression Therapy can be in evaluating and treating emotional and physical illness. Those of you with open minds will immediately see the value and understand the importance of incorporating such therapy into the medical evaluation and treatment of many conditions. Many lives could be saved by preventing suicides. Medical costs would be reduced by diagnosing a patient's condition sooner, thus eliminating the need for expensive, sophisticated testing, which would no longer be necessary.

For those of you who have not read my first book I would like to fill you in on how I began this unbelievable spiritual journey, or put in another way, how I, a medical doctor, reached beyond my conventionality to where my research took me and discovered my life's path in this rather negative and tumultuous world. Read on, I think you will enjoy and at the same time blow your mind discovering what I discovered.

Chapter 2

MY INTRODUCTION TO HYPNOSIS AND PAST LIFE REGRESSION

The year was 1990, and I was completing my 22nd year of practice in obstetrics and gynecology in Chardon, Ohio, a small town just outside of Cleveland. I decided to attend a course in medical hypnosis, purely out of curiosity, and was utterly impressed with its potential for healing. Following this course, I began to read books on past life regression by Dr. Brian Weiss and Roger Wolger. I was completely blown away by what I read and felt that I really wanted to do this. In my mind I could foresee a whole new way of approaching a patient's problem, one that could easily supplement conventional medical and surgical treatment. It would be a method that would bring a person's emotions to the forefront of his medical condition, thus allowing these emotions to be completely understood and integrated into the treatment plan. Unfortunately my Air Force Reserve squadron was activated for Desert Storm within that same month, and I found myself gone from practice for several months. This absence was not good for my practice but at least it was not a two-year stint, as was the case when I was drafted for the Viet Nam war.

TAKING THE PLUNGE

Upon returning from Desert Storm I decided to take the plunge and try out regression therapy on patients who were willing to do so. I thought I could accomplish this by carrying out hypnosis sessions after office hours and while waiting for patients in labor. This was feasible, since my office was adjacent to the hospital. I really wasn't sure how this would be accepted by my patients, but somehow I knew I had to give it a shot.

As it turned out, the patients that I approached in regard to carrying out these hypnotic regression sessions were extremely eager to undergo past life regression. I was not only pleasantly surprised, I was utterly astounded at the number of patients who displayed an open mind in regard to reincarnation. As I continued to regress more patients it became obvious that the results were unmistakably beneficial.

SYNCHRONICITY CAN FUEL ONE'S MOMENTUM

Once again the higher powers were showing me that everything happens for a reason. This took the form of being one of my earliest patients who agreed to undergo past life regression. She was a 48-year-old legal secretary by the name of Evelyn. Her problem was recurring nightmares that were becoming more frequent, causing her to wake up screaming. She also harbored phobias, including a fear of guns and horses.

Her several regressions under deep hypnosis were unbelievably vivid in their descriptions and emotional content. I was totally impressed with her ability to completely take on the persona of her previous lifetimes and truly become that person in voice and personality. She was able to see dates clearly in her mind, which revealed an uncanny accuracy when matched with historical events, allowing me to be able to validate 90% of her lifetimes. As if that were not impressive enough, this patient exhibited a phenomenon known as xenoglossy, the ability to speak a language not learned or known. In her life as a Druid High Priestess, she spoke ancient Gaelic. Following several sessions Evelyn ceased having nightmares and was cured of her phobias.

The intrinsic quality and timing of her regression sessions add credence to the old age truism that "things happen for a reason." This particular case was most certainly the impetus that propelled me well on my way to becoming passionate about past life regression therapy. As I saw more patients I began to feel as if I were tapping into the mysteries of the universe, answering questions such as who am I, where did I come from, why am I here, and where do I go when I leave this Earth?

My thirty-second year in practice became a milestone in my life. That year I developed severe cervical arthritis in my neck, a common ailment among surgeons and one which made me unable to carry out surgery and deliveries in a safe manner. This rather unfortunate situation forced me to make a decision I'll never regret. In the year 2000 I decided to leave the cold, wet Ohio weather and retire to the warm, dry climate of Las Vegas. After a few months in Las Vegas my arthritic symptoms magically abated, and I thrust myself completely into research on past life regression.

THE JOURNEY BEGINS

I learned that Dr. Raymond Moody, the Father of the Near Death Experience, was conducting Consciousness classes at the University of Nevada in Las Vegas. I had communicated with him 31 years earlier about a case that I had, and found out that he was quite knowledgeable and was on a quest involving extensive research on near-death experiences. When I called him, he remembered me and asked what I was doing. My research was rather interesting to him, and he invited me to give lectures to his class regarding my work. This opened the door and led to a treasure trove of experience when

I called for volunteer students to undergo gratis regression sessions for my research. The massive amount of appointments for regression kept me busy for at least two years. This included Dr. Moody's students, their friends, and their relatives. My research began to take on a life of its own as I soon began to see marked improvement in the subjects undergoing hypnotic regression.

The many subjects that I had seen had many reasons for undergoing past life regression. Here are just some of those reasons:

- To explain the causes of phobias, fears, and hang-ups
- To understand why you feel connected to certain people
- To clear out obstructions to joy and happiness in your present life
- To gain insight into the lessons you need to learn in this life
- To explain your preferences for certain cultures, places, or time periods in history
- To find out what other talents you may have had in other lives
- To no longer fear death by understanding that you are an eternal being
- To explain déjà vu
- Curiosity

LOVE THOSE SPIRIT GUIDES

Occasionally a patient under hypnosis would mention seeing or feeling the presence of his Spirit Guide. This made me recall a patient that I had seen for many years in my OB/GYN practice. She had not returned for at least four years, but when she finally made a GYN appointment, her condition was such that it demanded that I carry out an exploratory laparotomy as soon as possible. Upon opening her abdomen it became obvious that she had a fulminating advanced intestinal cancer. Breaking the news to her was among the most difficult tasks that I had to perform as a physician. I felt that a past life regression session would help her cope with this unbelievably depressing situation. As it turned out, the regression experience was very beneficial. Seeing herself dying and being reborn over and over helped her to know without any reservations that she is an eternal being, and her soul lives on forever as it sheds its temporal physical body from lifetime to lifetime. Thus she was able to achieve inner peace, a sense of being eternal, and a whole different way of looking at life and death, something every dying person needs to experience.

One of her lifetimes was as a nurse's helper in a large tent serving as a makeshift Confederate hospital close to the battle that was raging at Gettysburg. After advancing her in time and eventually through the death experience, she entered the Light. While in the afterlife I asked her what she had learned in this lifetime. She replied, "I learned the importance of comforting those with great suffering." She then said that she will soon be helping someone on Earth, but as yet did not know the identity of that person. She is to be a protector, a Spirit Guide.

Dick Sutphen, president of the American Board of Hypnotherapy since 2007 and author of a great number of excellent books, including the million-copy reincarnation bestseller, *You Were Born Again To Be Together*, was one of the earliest and greatest pioneers in past life regression therapy. He would often take a subject up to his Higher Self hypnotically and have the subject telepathically communicate with his own Spirit Guide. Dick Sutphen also wrote a book about Spirit Guides entitled, *With Your Spirit Guide's Help*. With this in mind I decided to routinely have the patients ascend hypnotically to their Higher Self and then call for their Spirit Guide. I would then make good use of the Spirit Guide by communicating directly with him or her through the patient, a form of channeling. I would start off by asking the Spirit Guide's name and if he or she would be willing to help me resolve the patient's problems. The answers would come into the patient's mind telepathically, allowing the patient to answer. I would then ask many questions such as, how long have you been with the patient. Have you had any lifetimes with him? How many lifetimes has the patient had? Has the patient had any parallel lifetimes? Parallel lives are believed to occur when the soul divides and occupies two or more bodies so as to learn lessons from different perspectives. According to my subjects and their Spirit Guides, the same soul can occupy more than one body during an incarnation or in overlapping incarnations. I also ask the Spirit Guide if the patient has had lifetimes in Atlantis or on other planets, and so on.

My many years of experience in communicating with Spirit Guides have yielded the following information that I feel I should share. I have found Spirit Guides to be non-physical beings who were mostly living human beings at one time. Occasionally I have encountered a Spirit Guide who was from another planet. Following their death as humans they choose to volunteer or are assigned to one or more human beings for the purpose of helping and guiding them. Spirit Guides are not attached and therefore do not draw energy from the person they are helping. They come from the Light and thus have their own source of energy. They are very humanistic and have very specific personalities. Some are humorous, others are all business; most of them, however, are very cooperative. Personality traits such as humor and irritability seem to be present even in the spirit realm. During one session I was admonished by the patient's Spirit Guide for asking too many questions and told that I was diverting energy from its proper place. In another case I was told that the patient is not ready and that it would not be in the patient's best interest to revisit certain lifetimes at this time. I was, however, given a go-ahead to proceed with an exploration of those lives in the patient's third session.

Some guides are exceptionally wise and very helpful; others are not, and when I feel that I'm not accomplishing what I need to, I'll ask for another Spirit Guide with more experience to step forward. On occasion I've even called for a third Spirit Guide. During one of my sessions I witnessed a Spirit Guide's panic reaction during the removal of a large group of dark force entities, described as "legions of dark forces." The Spirit Guide screamed, "There are too many of them!" This case will be discussed in detail later in this book.

My research has shown that there are many Spirit Guides assigned to each person, some of whom specialize in helping during specific situations. One of the Guides will usually come forth when called upon during the altered state of consciousness encountered while under deep hypnosis. I routinely ask the patient to tell me if he can see, hear, or otherwise sense the presence of the energy of his Spirit Guide. In my experience, I have found that patients respond positively to this question approximately 70-80% of the time. Occasionally the patient is unaware of the Spirit Guide's presence, however the Guide will still speak through the patient. Another 10-15% of the time, the Spirit Guide is unattainable, and in the majority of these cases the patient cannot be regressed. This situation caused me great concern since I was becoming accustomed to and enjoying working with Spirit Guides. As my experience with Spirit Guides increased I realized that I was gaining an enormous amount of information about them; however, I felt that finding the reason for this inability to obtain one's Spirit Guide would be one of my main goals.

Several months after arriving in Las Vegas I received a phone call from Evelyn, my former patient from Ohio whose regressions were unbelievably vivid and verifiable. She even spoke ancient languages under hypnosis which I also validated. She told me that she had a conscious flashback of a life with me in the 12th century. I was a French knight, and she was my half-sister. As a French nobleman I was responsible for the security of my village, however the security was reduced considerably following my departure for the Crusades with my knights and practically nil when I and many of my knights did not return. Within the same year my archenemy, an evil Count from another part of France, invaded and destroyed my chateau and village, leaving only a handful of survivors, including my half-sister. My shield in that life bore my heraldry, which was a silver cross with alternating black and red colors and a rampant lion at the center of the cross.

I filed this information in the back of my mind as I reviewed this patient's chart and wished that I had begun using Spirit Guides at that time. If I had, I'm sure I would have attained a wealth of information regarding the life that I shared with this patient.

THE SPIRIT GUIDE EXPERIMENT

Spirit Guides had become such an inherent part of my work and yes— even my life— that I decided to somehow prove that these Guides were truly credible and authentic. Thus I designed an experimental model wherein I would ask nine individual Spirit Guides the same question, "Can you see my Spirit Guide? And if so, please describe his or her appearance." Eight of the nine Guides described my Spirit Guide as a medieval knight, and the ninth was close. Some of these descriptions were given in a brief manner, and others in great detail. Seven volunteered that he was in a medieval battle with me, stepped in front of me, and took a deathblow for me. When I asked the Guides to please describe me in that lifetime, several of them said that I was a French knight with a shield that had a silver cross, red and black colors, and a lion, just as my former patient Evelyn had described when she called me three years earlier in regard to her conscious flashback regarding her memories of a medieval life that we had shared. I had not spoken to her for several years so I decided to get in touch with her once again and tell her about the Spirit Guide experiment. I barely told her who was calling when she immediately interrupted me and said that she just had to tell me about a dream she had two nights ago. She said it was very lucid and quite real. It seems that a spirit in medieval armor visited her and said he was my Spirit Guide. He told her that he had been a French nobleman who joined forces with me during the long march to the Crusades. We became close and made a mutual pact to protect each other in the Holy War. He later took a deathblow in battle that was meant for me. I was completely shocked by what she had to say. In my mind I was now convinced that Spirit Guides are extremely real and credible and also the life that I shared with my Spirit Guide and my former patient, Evelyn, had indeed occurred.

CONVERTING GRIEF INTO PEACE

Losing someone you love is one of the most difficult experiences a human being can endure. When a patient's eyes begin to tear as he tells you about losing a loved one, you cannot help but feel his pain. I have experienced such empathy whenever a patient informs me that he or she has lost a spouse, a fiancé, a lover, a child, a parent, a sibling, or even a pet. It doesn't really matter how long ago the loss occurred. Grief and the heart-wrenching emotions that pour forth when the loved one died cause this memory to remain painfully prominent in both the conscious and the subconscious mind. When the patient comes to the realization that this loved one is no longer present in this physical world and that memories of that loved one are all he has left, he begins to understand that the one he loved so much is truly gone, permanently absent, and never to be seen on Earth again, leaving a very huge void in his life.

I have found that when I am working with patients who have had such losses, it is a great comfort for them to know that the loved one they miss so much is doing well. In order to accomplish this, I take the patient into deep hypnosis and have him imagine that he is walking into a beautiful garden with colorful and majestic flowers and waterfalls. I then have him sit on a large white marble bench and tell him that someone he loves and misses may come by and sit next to him on this bench. I instruct the patient to let me know if he sees someone coming, and then I just wait and remain silent for a short while. Within minutes the patient will either start sobbing or say, "I see someone coming." I will inquire as to who is there with him, and I will always see a smile through the tears when the patient tells me his loved one is here, the loved one usually appears in his prime if he was older at death, and as a young adult if he was a child.

I utilized this technique prior to my making good use of Spirit Guides, however since I began using the Guides I can also just ask them to please have the patient's deceased loved one visit him. The effect is identical without the frills of a garden, namely removing sadness and sorrow and replacing it with unmitigated joy and a knowing that this loved one is all right. Regardless of the technique used, sessions such as these give the patient the strength to accept such a loss and understand that this passing is a normal part of one's reincarnation cycle and that we are all eternal spirits who choose when to incarnate into this world. This moving experience leaves the patient feeling much more peaceful and more spiritual. This Spirit Guide shortcut comes in handy when I have an extreme amount of work to accomplish in one session.

Losing a son or daughter at any age is rough enough, however losing one at a young age is devastating. I recently had such a case. It involved a family from Quebec, Canada, who lost their five-year-old son, James, the younger of two children. James had aspirated part of a walnut and was hospitalized for several days after developing pneumonia, which soon took his life. His family was devastated.

James's mother called me two months after his death and asked if she could make contact with the spirit world under hypnosis and communicate with her son James. I told her that I had done this successfully many times and agreed to see her. When she arrived she was exceptionally nervous and very tearful when relaying what happened to James. I was finally able to calm her down and relax her enough so her hypnotic induction would be successful. I was then able to deepen her trance, take her up to her Higher Self, and call for her Spirit Guide, who did not come forward. I then decided to take her into a garden and see if we could have her deceased son visit with her. Unfortunately, this attempt at having James visit with his mother was unsuccessful. I then took the patient into a past lifetime and finally through a death experience and her entrance into the Light, at which time her Spirit Guide did come forward. Spirit Guides often come through when the patient is in the Light. The Spirit Guide was very helpful and said that James could not appear to his mother because he was attached to her.

Following this revelation I communicated with James, the attached spirit, who then told me that he wanted very much to be with his family. The Spirit Guide explained that being attached was not the answer; however, if he goes to the Light he will be able to continue his spiritual journey and will be in a position to incarnate and therefore may even join his family again by entering the body of a new baby when and if his mother again becomes pregnant. James agreed, and I helped him get to the Light. The patient's Spirit Guide confirmed that James was in the Light and predicted that he will return to his family in this way. I've seen many of these situations and have felt the pain that the parent carries in his or her heart.

Losing a spouse can sometimes put the remaining spouse into a deep depression or cause other emotional problems. One such case comes to mind. It involved a retired physician by the name of Steven, who lost his wife of well over 50 years. Her serious illness eventually put her in a hospital on life support in an unconscious state. Steven was forced to make that fateful decision to let her go by withdrawing all life support, leaving her on morphine alone. Miraculously, she awakened a few hours before she died. Steven felt the need to tell her she was dying and heard her reply, "I don't want to die." Following this statement she slipped back into a coma and died within a short time. Steven was devastated and fraught with guilt.

When I saw Steven as a patient, his wife had been dead for several years, and he was living with a woman who had also been a friend of his wife. This situation added to his feelings of guilt. Under deep hypnosis, the spirit of Steven's wife came to him, and they spoke for several minutes. Later Steven told me that his wife was doing well on her spiritual journey, and not only did she forgive him, but she understood why it was necessary for him to make that decision about removing her life support. She also gave him her blessing in regard to his relationship with her longtime friend. Steven left that session with an entirely different attitude, no longer feeling the pangs of guilt from pulling the plug on his wife's life support. In later sessions I took Steven back to many lifetimes that he had with both his wife and his lady friend. Steven died a few years later at the age of 90. I am sure he was quite happy to be with his wife again.

Another case had to do with an intelligent and loving father who lost his 24-year-old son several years earlier. After an emotional visit with the spirit of his son, the patient said that his son was doing okay and seemed older and wiser. In addition, the patient's son told his father, "Tell Mother not to worry, and we will all be together again."

REVIEWING MY BAPTISM OF FIRE

One of my research patients by the name of Jason became my "baptism of fire" in regard to my accidentally discovering something very important that was missing in my hypnotic evaluation and treatment of patients. Jason was a writer who always had an interest in feudal Japanese culture but over the past three years had developed an obsessive passion for this culture which would interfere with his writing and cause him to argue with himself. The patient also found that times of stress would bring on recollections of anger and regret, which were somehow related to this passion. When the patient was hypnotically taken back to the cause of these feelings, he saw himself as the teenage son of a feudal Japanese farmer. In that life Jason had a burning desire to join the Emperor's army. His parents supplied him with bamboo armor because they could not afford much.

He soon found himself marching at night with the Emperor's army through a narrow gorge and felt extremely proud to be part of this elite force and as such was very happy. Suddenly he heard screaming and thunderous hoof beats as fierce warriors brandishing long spears charged through their lines. He and many others were the first to be run through by these heavy spears during this surprise attack. As he was dying in the mud, a heavy voice came out of the patient's mouth, shouting in an angry manner that he had marched but never fought, and that he had not achieved any glory. It then said, "I am angry, and Jason doesn't do what I tell him." What I was hearing, and the scenario that was unfolding, was truly shocking to me as I began to realize that I was not regressing Jason but rather an entity that was most likely within him.

My mind began to be barraged with many emotions and many questions as I put forth the question, "How long have you been with Jason?" This spirit responded by telling me that Jason was a little boy when he joined him.

My mind was now in high gear as I began to realize that I was carrying on a conversation with a spirit of some sort, a discarnate being. By this time I had pretty much shed my conventionalism by carrying out past life regression therapy, but this mind-blowing situation was really way out there. I had very little experience in this area, however I remembered reading that the spirit of a person who dies and possesses another human being needs to go to the Light. As long as I was communicating with this spirit, I suggested that he ask for help from heavenly spirits to aid him in getting to the Light, where he will be able to continue his spiritual journey and be able to incarnate again. The attached entity finally agreed, and at that moment Jason said that he could feel this spirit leaving, and this made him feel much lighter. I then told Jason to say some prayers so as to protect him from further attachments.

As far as I'm concerned, this surprising and extraordinary experience opened up Pandora's Box and brought many questions to mind regarding regression therapy. On the other hand, it also appeared to open up many new vistas of hypnotic treatment that also held the promise of healing and led to extensive research with an intensive pursuit of knowledge regarding releasement of entities; and finally, to a decision to incorporate this form of therapy into my regression work. By doing so, I have learned much and I find that I am continuing to learn on a daily basis as I see patients; however I must admit that the knowledge that I have acquired regarding entity attachments is quite disturbing but at the same time is vital to the process of healing patients. I also have come to believe that releasing entities from patients should be a requirement for anyone who plans on conducting past life regression therapy.

TIME TO WRITE MY FIRST BOOK

The year was 2003, and the amount of material that I was amassing was of such proportions that I felt truly compelled to write my first book, *From Birth to Rebirth: Gnostic Healing for the 21st Century*. As I began to approach the organization of my notes and case studies I realized that this was going to be an imposing task. I decided to begin the book as an autobiography and talk about my feelings regarding medicine and my choice of specialties, namely OB/GYN. I then show how the transition from the conventional to the unconventional took place. The historical times and topics involved in the myriad of fascinating cases that I present touch upon ancient times, lost continents, future lives, man's first existence, lives on other planets, contact with extraterrestrials, and communication with attached entities and advanced spiritual beings, to name a few.

For those of you that have read my first book, I am sure that you began to understand my thoughts, my feelings, and yes, my unmitigated excitement as I continued to witness the influence of entity attachment and how highly emotional past life incidents were affecting and influencing a person's present life through negative subconscious programming of the conscious mind. As a physician I was able to envision the powerful healing potential of past life regression therapy and as such have influenced many physicians, some of whom have now come to me as patients.

When I wrote my first book I decided to give the reader some idea of what a person endures to become a physician. This included the stiff competition when one applies to medical school, the trials and tribulations one goes through in medical school, and what it's like to experience the challenges of internship and residency. One of the reasons I chose obstetrics and gynecology as my specialty was because my only sibling suffered a brain injury prior to birth due to nurses holding my mother's legs together so my sister wouldn't deliver until the physician arrived. The result was a severe form of cerebral palsy which has caused my sister great limitations and much distress throughout her life. I wanted to contribute to the best performance of that specialty as I possibly could. Following my residency I was drafted into the Air Force due to the Vietnam War, and two years later I was able to begin practice.

I talk about what it's like to safely deliver babies, carry out difficult surgeries, and go without sleep, all this so as to help the reader understand what it's like to be a conventional physician. I then describe how a physician can feel after twelve years of practice, with minimal sleep and a heavy load of patients, deliveries, and surgeries. The description was "burned out," and I needed something, so I decided to reactivate my Air Force commission and join the Reserve. I had another physician cover me so I could take time off to train to be a Flight Surgeon and very much enjoyed the excitement that I experienced during our training missions in the B-52 bombers and fighter trainers. As it turned out, experiencing this kind of excitement while serving my country was just what I needed to relieve the stress of day to day practice.

THE KARMIC MONKEY-WRENCH

I thought I had come to the point in my life where I considered myself exceptionally enlightened, and as such I had a firm belief that there were certain principles related to reincarnation and karma that were infallible and stood on their own merit, namely:

* We are responsible for our actions
* There are no victims
* Free will is involved in our every action
* We create our own reality

After many years of witnessing the unbelievable effects that attached entities have upon the patient/host, it became obvious that these entities represent the proverbial, disruptive, and inimical monkey-wrench that has been thrown into the basic precepts of reincarnation and karma. The startling result is:

* We may not always be responsible for our actions
* Some of us can become victims
* Our greatest gift, that of free will, can be interfered with
* We may not always be creating our own reality

You, the reader, may think you are your own person; you are calling your own shots; you are master of your own fate! I certainly did. But now I know that this is not always the case. Please bear in mind that everything coming from the patient's subconscious mind while under deep hypnosis *comes from the patient*, not from me. Thus far, my experience with releasement of entities coincides with the experience of pioneers in this field, namely the late Dr. William Baldwin and Dr. Edith Fiore. As the following pages unfold you will be able to witness an array of case histories, many of which will involve the presence of attached entities, with whom I have communicated through my patients. Many words can be used to describe the purpose of these entities in regard to joining their host: namely love, compassion, jealousy, revenge, drug and alcohol addictions; the list is endless.

As my hypnotherapy practice expanded, my exposure to various types of attached entities increased. I became convinced through personal experience that spiritual entities are indeed *real*. Though unaware of their presence, my patients displayed various negative effects of these attached entities which were very real and caused abnormal behavior. These detrimental effects involved the patients' physical, mental, and emotional states. Comprehensive Hypnoregression Therapy discovers the underlying cause of a patient's emotional or physical ailment by investigating the subconscious mind. The major causes of these problems are emotional past life memories and the influence of entities attached to the patient.

Comprehensive Hypnoregression Therapy is extremely successful. I would hope that conventional medical doctors will one day be open enough in their thinking to begin to understand that reincarnation is a true fact and realize that the experiences of many millions of people, who have had near death experiences, are almost identical to the descriptions of the death experience and afterlife by millions of people under regression. Throw in many thousands of regressions that have been validated and people speaking languages that are unknown to them, and you have massive evidence of reincarnation. And yes, these testimonies also show us a proof of sorts—that our consciousness continues on following physical death, and one's soul moves to a spiritual dimension where other souls reside. Hypnotic regression and near death experiences have given us a definite glimpse into this etheric dimension of spirit energy. Should we ignore these gifts that help answer the eternal questions about who we are, what we are doing here, and where we go when we leave? I think not. Skeptics will always take an affront to this way of thinking and insist that we need to prove these things scientifically. I feel that such scientific methods are part and parcel of the physical realm that humans live in and cannot easily be used to prove spiritual matters; however, the future may prove me to be wrong.

Chapter 3

ATTACHED ENTITIES

My research has yielded results which are similar to the work of the late Dr. William Baldwin, namely that these different types of entities are both human and non-human, and that I am able to communicate with these entities in the same way as I do with Spirit Guides. I ask questions of these entities, and the answers come in to the patient's mind and are communicated to me through the patient. My experience with Spirit Guides is that the majority of them were in a human body at one time, and some even had lifetimes with the patient. Also, I have encountered Spirit Guides who were extraterrestrials. I therefore feel that Spirit Guides can be human or non-human. I have also had experience with many of the categories that Dr. Baldwin speaks of, and I will touch upon some of these cases, but for the most part I intend to dwell upon the most common entities that I have found to be most responsible for affecting the patient in a negative way. I refer the reader to Dr. Baldwin's textbook, *Spirit Releasement Therapy*, for a detailed description of these less-common entities. A rarely encountered entity that I found most interesting is an inter-dimensional being, and I discuss two such cases in Chapter Seven.

The most common human entities that I personally have encountered include:

* Earthbound spirit attachments which are disembodied human spirits. They are the consciousness that survives after a person dies. These spirits decline going to the Light and join a living person for various reasons, thus allowing the physical and emotional problems that existed when they were alive to affect the patient/host.
* Mind or soul fragments which are fragmentations of a living person's consciousness that have separated from that individual and did not return but rather attached to another person. The fragmentation is usually a result of traumatic circumstances. Their emotional and physical problems can also affect the patient/host.
* Terminated pregnancies
* Spirit Guides (unless they are extraterrestrial). They are not attached and do not draw energy from the person they are helping with guidance.

The most common non-human attached entities that I have encountered include:

* Extraterrestrial beings and their implants
* Dark force entities (My medieval life as a French knight included an evil French nobleman who became a powerful dark force in the hierarchy of the dark forces. This appears to be an exception to the theory that all dark forces are non-human. (See Chapter Five, *The Powerful Dark Force Entity Who Knows Me.*)

My research also shows that entities who were once human seem to imprint their personality quirks and their emotional and physical ailments upon the host, whereas non-human entities are there for the purpose of completing their agenda. Many times a patient's issues are due to the effects of both types of entities. In addition, all attached entities are drawing energy from their host.

THE IMPORTANCE OF RELEASING ATTACHED ENTITIES

My techniques in discovering and identifying entities and diagnosing their effects on the patient/host differ somewhat from Dr. Baldwin's methods in that I utilize the patient's Spirit Guide to a great extent. In doing so I have found that most of these Guides have had human lifetimes on Earth, some with the patient, and even some in the patient's present lifetime.

As I began to incorporate and integrate entity releasement therapy into my past life regression sessions, I immediately saw no reason why I could not ask the Spirit Guide about the presence of foreign energy and felt that this methodology would expedite the process. This evolved into delineating the types and numbers of attached entities present and having a Spirit Guide monitor and report on the progress of the various steps involved during the releasement of entities. This was especially helpful during an exorcism of dark force entities (getting rid of dark forces), and more importantly, I was able to obtain confirmation of each entity being released and taken to designated destinations, no longer attached to the patient and no longer in a position to reattach or to attach to someone else. My intuition was telling me that combining entity releasement with past life regression therapy would definitely have an impact on the success rate of the sessions. I just didn't realize how much.

Here I am discussing the removal of spirits and the exorcism of dark-force entities, something I couldn't even conceive of doing when I was in practice delivering babies and performing surgery. Yet I find that my spiritual enlightenment has taken me to this point in my life for a reason, and I feel it is a very good reason. My main thrust has always been to help people with physical and emotional problems and cure them if possible. Well, past life regression therapy, along with entity releasement therapy, is allowing me to do just that. The result is an unbelievable increase in the cure rate of patients, so much so that I am now of the mind that if one is to conduct past life regression therapy, one must also carry out releasement of entities, the combination of which I have come to call Comprehensive

Hypnoregression Therapy. I have thus come to the conclusion that a patient's emotional or physical problem is often related to one of two causes or a combination of the two. The first cause is a highly emotional past life memory that has been triggered and brought to the surface of the subconscious mind by something or someone in the patient's present life. Once this has occurred it can easily program the patient's conscious mind in a very negative way and cause needless suffering.

The second cause has to do with the presence of an attached entity who is able to adversely affect the patient in many ways. These entities are uninvited, work through other dimensions, and draw energy from the patient/host. Most patients are completely unaware of the causes of their suffering until the conscious mind, which is fully awake during hypnosis, observes and understands what the subconscious mind reveals. The multitude of effects upon the patient/host, by various forms of entity attachments, will be described in detail in case histories that will follow.

THE NECESSITY OF NAILING DOWN THE CAUSE

Hypnotherapy is extremely helpful when one needs to rid himself of harmful habits, the most common of which are smoking and overeating. The dangers involved with such habits are quite obvious and can easily lead to serious medical conditions which may result in death. As usual, human emotions play a big part in perpetuating the continuation of such habits. People will often smoke or overeat due to emotional stress, and some individuals push the envelope by smoking three to four packs of cigarettes per day or by becoming morbidly obese. I had encountered all of the above in my early years of medical practice and wish I knew then what I know now in regard to helping people with such problems. I had to perform emergency surgery on patients such as this on many occasions and yes, the harmful habits that brought on the patient's high risk medical condition were now responsible for increasing the risks of surgery and causing the case to be more complicated and a greater challenge for both the surgeon and the anesthesiologist.

In order to have you, the reader, obtain a greater understanding of what an OB/GYN physician goes through when a patient does push the envelope with the harmful habit of overeating, I'd like to give you a view of morbid obesity from a physician's perspective. I am now retired from my OB/GYN practice and no longer have to face these problems, however I feel sorry for my younger colleagues who are now feeling even more stress from complications of obese pregnant women and obese GYN patients, which I understand has now increased. Statistics show:

* Obesity is common, serious, and costly. In 2011-2012, more than one-third of U.S. adults (34.9%) were obese.
* In 2011-2012, approximately 17%, of children and adolescents aged 2—19 years were obese.
* Obesity-related conditions include heart disease, stroke, type 2 diabetes and certain types of cancer. These are some of the leading causes of preventable death.[7]

I have had many obese patients in my 32+ years of practice and entirely too many morbidly obese patients. These cases were night-marish and often reminded me of an engineering project. One such case involved a short and very wide 465 pound woman, who required a D & C to rule out cancer. The mechanical equipment required to lift her onto a table with stirrups was of no value since the table was much too narrow for her gigantic torso. I attempted to do the D & C in a hospital bed but soon found that it was impossible to get to her vaginal vault, even with several people helping to retract her legs and thighs. In this situation, courage and valor took a back seat to safety, so I finally told the anesthesiologist to wake her up from the very light and very careful anesthesia they were using. The

---

7 [http://www.cdc.gov/obesity/data/adult.html#Costly], April 29, 2015

anesthesiologist was overjoyed at the prospect of ending the procedure, as his job was as dangerous as mine. The patient was sent to a large University hospital that had bigger surgical tables and larger lifts. I remember that patient very well. Her specially constructed wheelchair was exceptionally large, very strong, and very much needed, since she was unable to walk due to the obesity.

Abdominal surgery on morbidly obese women was also fraught with an array of potential complications. Another case that remains permanently imprinted in my mind was a 385-pound obstetric patient in labor, who required an immediate emergency Caesarian section because of having an abruptio placentae (premature separation of a normally implanted placenta [afterbirth] from the uterus). This diagnosis was made when the patient exhibited fetal cardiac distress (abnormalities of the baby's heartbeat), impending maternal shock (mother's blood pressure dropping), and increasing tenderness and tightening of the uterus.

Prenatal care was difficult enough, but I knew surgery was not going to be a picnic. Intravenous fluids and blood were immediately started, and following the induction of general anesthesia by a very nervous anesthesiologist, I decided to make a midline abdominal incision in this very obese abdomen. Normally I try to use a pfannenstiel (low horizontal) incision, however this patient had a history of pelvic inflammatory disease in her younger days, and I was extremely concerned about running into excessive pelvic adhesions (tissues and organs densely adherent to each other). The midline incision would also give me more options to open the uterus safely without damaging the bowel, the bladder, large blood vessels, and ureters (tubes connecting the bladder to the kidneys). It also would allow me the room to do a hysterectomy if we had to. Occasionally it is necessary to remove the uterus in cases of abruptio placentae.

The excessive adipose (fat) tissue prevented heavy bleeding while the midline abdominal incision was being carried out through at least six to seven inches of abdominal fat tissue. Bleeding remained relatively light after I entered the abdominal cavity and carefully took down the bladder flap that covered the lower uterine area. This surgery presented an unbelievable challenge as I had to delicately separate densely adherent tissues in a careful but rapid fashion, since I was also in a race against time. I needed to get this large, compromised infant delivered and on oxygen before his fetal distress took its toll. At the same time I knew that the rapidity of the surgery had to be tempered with a meticulous dissection of the adhesions so as not to endanger the mother. When I cut through the uterus using a horizontal lower uterine segment incision, a perfuse amount of blood poured forth from the uterine sinuses (dilated channels or receptacles containing chiefly venous blood) that had remained open after the placenta (afterbirth) prematurely separated. Also, excessive amounts of blood was squirting out from several large blood vessels which had been severed by opening the uterus. Suctioning by my assistant was ongoing but minimally helpful in that deep hole I was working in. My heart was racing as I widened the incision with my fingers, ruptured the bag of waters, and reached deeply for the baby's head. Delivering the limp body of the baby, we quickly clamped and cut the umbilical cord and handed the baby off to the pediatrician, who immediately suctioned and resuscitated the infant. I had my hands full delivering the placenta and stopping the massive bleeding by squeezing the uterus into a tight ball as the anesthesiologist started more blood and intravenous Pitocin (medication that tightens the uterus.) Tightening the uterus in this way closes the venous sinuses and slows the bleeding down dramatically. I then sutured the uterine incision, which was also bleeding excessively. Working in this very deep cavity forced me to use specially made, very long instruments, including clamps and suture holders. The venous sinuses and the edges of the uterine incision began to bleed more heavily, since the uterus was not tightening down as it should. I am sure this was related to the patient's obesity. In order to clamp these bleeders, I needed a certain degree of leverage which was difficult to achieve with these extra-long instruments. Also, the profuse bleeding continued to obstruct my vision in spite of vigorous suctioning by my assistants. I decided to once again manually tighten the uterus. This slowed the bleeding somewhat, and I was able to clamp the vigorous bleeders on the uterine incision. Once the extreme bleeding was finally stopped, I began to breathe easier and told my team to relax and allow the tension in the room to dissipate.

The baby and mother did fine; however the doctor, yours truly, like most obstetricians, drove himself home that morning bedraggled from no sleep and lots of stress, but still feeling good about the outcome in spite of complications like morbid obesity, over which he has very little control.

We must stop the spiraling increase in obesity that is showing up every day and is contributing to serious illnesses such as elevated blood pressure, diabetes, and other dangerous conditions. Proper eating is all very helpful, as well as exercise; however, it is imperative that hypnotic past life regression and entity releasement therapy be integrated into conventional medicine so as to treat these people in a proper and exceptionally successful way. Once again I reiterate it is absolutely necessary to nail down the cause of the patient's problem and then flood his subconscious mind with the right suggestions to eliminate this form of self-destructive behavior completely. Utilizing what I have learned will help the patients do just this.

What I do now is beyond the standard hypnotherapeutic approach, which mostly uses powerful suggestions to the patient's subconscious mind. I firmly believe that the subconscious mind is also the path that takes the therapist to the cause of the patient's obesity, which now can be exposed to the very observant conscious mind of the patient, which will understand and make judgments in regard to both past life events or attached entities that have contributed to the obesity. The use of Comprehensive Hypnoregression, which includes entity releasement, has proven itself time and time again, by curing most people of their physical and emotional problems. Such therapy will definitely increase the cure rate of obesity and prevent relapse to a much greater degree than standard hypnotherapy.

Often, emotional reactions to stress in one's current life will add to the problem and reinforce the cause of the obesity or other detrimental habits, such as smoking. If this is the case, the patient will often seek relief by emotional eating or sucking on a cigarette, both of which could be throwbacks to one's infancy that allowed these reactions to provide emotional comfort.

I have had a morbidly obese patient who was asked under hypnosis to go back to the cause of her obesity. After a few moments her face took on a painful grimace as she saw herself as a man dying of starvation over a long period of time in a Nazi concentration camp during World War II. I have also seen a patient who, when asked to go to the cause of her obesity, saw herself trying to survive a bitter cold winter in the great northwest and being unable to hunt for or gather food successfully. In that lifetime she died a cruel death of slow starvation. Some patients have had more than one life where they died of starvation. Something in their present lifetime acts as a trigger to bring these highly emotional prominent memories to the surface of the subconscious mind so that even minimal feelings of hunger will cause these powerful past life emotions to flood the patient's conscious mind and bring on the emotional overeating.

On several occasions I have uncovered subconscious reasons that a patient chooses to remain obese. One of those reasons was to be as unattractive as possible. One such patient would look or feel attractive from time to time and subsequently find herself becoming bombarded by a subconscious memory of a past life where being very beautiful caused her to be a victim of a brutal rape. Once the patient's conscious mind sees and understands what the subconscious has brought forth, it is able to release the effect, making powerful suggestions that follow much more effective. I have also seen several patients who had attached Earthbound spirits who had emotional eating problems of their own in their lifetime and were imprinting these problems onto the patient/host. Once these entities were identified and released into the Light, the influence upon the patient/host was nullified and suggestions to the subconscious became more meaningful.

In regard to smoking, I have seen many patients stop smoking after releasing Earthbound spirits who were heavy chain smokers. I have also had patients who had past lifetimes as a smoker, one as a chronic pipe smoker in the 1800s and another as a chain cigarette smoker in the 1940s. As I mentioned earlier, the suggestions that I instill regarding smoking are extremely helpful. One of those suggestions is that if the patient were ever to put a cigarette in his mouth again, it would taste like burning rubber. I mention this because one of my patients sent me an email several weeks after her session, saying that she had not smoked since she saw me, however she was very curious about what I had said about putting a cigarette in her mouth and just had to see if the cigarette would really taste like burning rubber. It did!

THE VOLUNTEER SPIRIT GUIDE

I normally put a lot of effort into getting the Spirit Guide to come forth. If the initial call for the Spirit Guide fails, I then regress the patient into a past life and through the death experience. Once the patient's soul is in the afterlife I once again have the patient call for the Spirit Guide. This technique is often successful. When it isn't, I will call for a certain volunteer Spirit Guide by the name of Abel. Some time ago Abel introduced himself to me as one of my patient's Spirit Guides. I was very impressed with Abel and soon discovered that he was very close to becoming a Master Spirit. I decided to ask for his advice in regard to the problem I had been encountering in getting a Spirit Guide to come forth. This problem occurred in roughly ten to fifteen percent of patients and often appeared to be associated with the patient also not being able to be regressed. I told Abel that I suspected that the dark forces were responsible. Abel immediately interrupted and said, "You're correct. The dark forces are keeping the Spirit Guide from coming forth and preventing the patient from entering a past life."

I asked, "How does this happen?"

Abel replied, "The dark forces and especially the more powerful dark force entities create a fog-like mist which prevents the guide from coming through."

I then asked, "What can I do about it?"

His answer was, "Call me."

Abel has come through to help monitor the presence and releasement of attached entities at least 550 or more times. However there still have been many occasions, approximately 20% of the times he has been called, when Abel could not get through to help. In one of those cases the patient heard a voice saying, "You're not getting through." Most patients see Abel as a beam of light; however, I have had many patients describe him in more detail, and they made special mention of the fact that he had a red beard.

THE GOD LIGHT VISUALIZATION AND AFFIRMATION

When I have successfully removed all foreign energy from a patient and have received confirmation from a true Spirit Guide, I will instruct the patient in carrying out a God Light visualization and an affirmation which will be a tremendous help in avoiding future attachments. This endeavor places spiritual armor upon the patient, who then lets these intrusive entities, especially the dark forces, know who he is, namely a spiritual being that lives forever and carries the Light of God within him. By repeating this visualization the patient is in effect saying, "I am the Captain of my Soul and no, I do not want you uninvited parasitic infestations in my space. The Light of God radiates through my entire being and surrounds me with God Light protection which will maintain the harmony of my true being."

The God Light Visualization is as follows:

The Creator has placed within me a knowing that I carry a part of God within me. It is the Light of God's love in the form of a spark that ignites and explodes, filling every subatomic particle within my being and every space that was or could be occupied by foreign energy. This golden white violet light extends beyond my body and surrounds me as a protective shield.

I have the patient promise that he will carry out this God Light Visualization upon waking, before meals, and before going to sleep. Once a person understands what to visualize, it is not necessary to repeat these words. All that is needed is to picture a spark of God Light within you, exploding, filling your body and surrounding you with a protective shield of God Light. This visualization can be completed in a matter of a few seconds. It is very similar to the Sealing Light Meditation that Dr. William Baldwin wrote about in his books.

The Affirmation that I encourage patients to use was given to me by Jim Nichols, a UFO researcher, historian, and world renowned illustrator who I found to be exceptionally intelligent and very spiritually enlightened. The Affirmation is as follows, to be carried out in the morning and in the evening and whenever a negative thought comes to mind:

"The Light of God never fails," to be repeated three times;
"I live this day in God Light," to be repeated three times;
And, finally, "The harmony of my true being is my ultimate protection," said once.

HOW I CONDUCT MY SESSIONS

My initial interview with patients includes informing them how I use terms like sleep, deep sleep, and trance; however, I let them know that their conscious mind is always fully awake and aware of everything that occurs. I explain that I am having the patient enter an altered state of consciousness which resembles sleep but is not sleep, and that I do this by relaxing him with my voice and thus lower his brain wave frequency from "beta," the waking state beyond "alpha," the meditative state, to "theta," the hypnotic state, which is just above "delta," the sleeping state. I let the patient know that he is always in control; that will power is not compromised, and that a strong willed person makes an even better subject. I also tell the patient to concentrate on what I am saying and not think other thoughts, such as, "I just heard an airplane going over; I don't think I'm under hypnosis."

I also make it clear to the patients that they really do not want their conscious mind to interfere with the process by analyzing, questioning, or criticizing what's happening. In other words, the patient should go with the flow. I tell the patient to listen only to what I am saying and the sound of the music in the background. My explanations of the hypnotic process include the fact that the background music carries a theta brainwave frequency, which is also of help during the induction of this hypnotic altered state of con- sciousness. While in this hypnotic state, the patient remains physi- cally relaxed and mentally concentrated as the subconscious mind is allowed to surface and become suggestible to suggestions that are acceptable and at the same time be able to retrieve prominent emo- tional memories long since forgotten by the conscious mind.

All hypnosis is self-hypnosis. The patient must be cooperative and motivated and understand that he can refuse suggestions that he may find to be unacceptable. There are no dangers involved if the patient is not a threat to himself or others. If a patient were to be left alone while in the hypnotic state, he would wake up on his own or fall asleep and then wake up.

Once the patient is under deep hypnosis, I take him up to his Higher Self and have him call for a Spirit Guide to help. Once a Spirit Guide comes forth, I will ask if he or she will accept the gift of light. If I get an affirmative answer, and I feel this Spirit Guide is valid, I will then ask if he will assist me in helping the patient with his problems. I then ask if the patient has any foreign energy, and if dark forces are present, I will conduct an immediate exorcism. I will then interrogate the remaining foreign energy in regard to the patient's issues before sending them away to appropriate destinations. The Spirit Guide helps with every step of the way during the removal of foreign energy and confirms that they have arrived at specific destinations. The Spirit Guide will help conduct a soul retrieval if the patient's soul has been fragmented and then is asked if past life memories have contributed to the patient's problems. If so, he is then asked to take us to each memory that's involved so the patient can fully understand and release the negative effect of the memory. The session usually will come to an end after the patient receives advice from his Spirit Guide, is taught protective measures, and powerful suggestions are given to solidify his improved status.

One can easily see how Comprehensive Hypnoregression Therapy allows this healing to take place through the awesome power of the mind by having the subconscious mind take center stage within the spotlight so it may allow the Spirit Guide to check for foreign energy frequencies and later bring up the memory of the events from past lives that are causing problems for the patient. At the same time, the conscious mind finds itself in a front row seat in the audience where it can observe what the subconscious mind brings forth. If the patient's problem was due to an attached entity, the patient will understand that the problem will improve when the entity is removed. If the patient's problem is due to an emotional memory of a past life event, the patient's conscious mind will make a distinction of time and then a judgment that this event happened a long time ago and has no relationship to the patient's present life and therefore its effect on the patient will be released.

How powerful is the mind? It is unbelievably powerful; it can even alter cellular growth. Most researchers will tell you that we only use 10% of our brain. I feel very strongly that Comprehensive

Hypnoregression Therapy, utilizing both the conscious and the subconscious mind, will one day be the key to unlock the mystery of how powerful the mind is, and this will benefit all mankind beyond our wildest dreams. The potential of hypnotic healing has been too long ignored. Its abomination as stage entertainment needs to end so it can be recognized for what it rightfully is: an exceptional healing modality in medicine.

Hypnotherapy is very successful in treating anxiety, depression, insomnia, fears, phobias, habits, addictions, and many more undesirable and hurtful conditions. If one incorporates Comprehensive Hypnoregression techniques into such therapy, the percent of patients cured of emotional and physical problems increases dramatically, and the reason for this is that one's subconscious mind is an endless reservoir of detailed memories of every life he has ever lived. These memories affect his personality, his thoughts, and his physical and emotional responses to everything that enters his consciousness. Moreover, the subconscious mind is the portal through which the Comprehensive Hypnoregression therapist is able to communicate with the patient's Spirit Guide and attached entities.

My sessions were–and still are–lasting two and a half to three hours. My experience with a great number of patients has become my reality, and it has greatly contributed to my research on the doctrines of reincarnation and karma and on the release of entity attachments. I feel very strongly that such doctrines and entities are extremely real, but I truly believe that we will not know how it all works until we are in the spiritual dimension. I therefore have a great disdain for comments from "authorities" who say, "This is how it is." We are always learning, and I for one have learned a great deal from my patients, and as such have been able to fit many of the pieces of the puzzle together, however I will be the first to admit that we have barely scratched the surface. In Chapter Seventeen I will elaborate even further on how I feel these sessions should be carried out.

DUAL HYPNOSIS

If I am unable to get a Spirit Guide or the volunteer Spirit Guide Abel, I will strongly suspect dark forces and will try to get them to show themselves by calling them out. Occasionally I will get a response to my confrontation such as, "You're not strong enough."

I thought long and hard about the many instances when Abel could not get through and regression was not possible, so I ended up devising another way to use a volunteer Spirit Guide, but this time it would be through another subject during the same hypnotic session, with the patient and the volunteer subject on separate couches. I called this approach "dual hypnosis."

I would often have a husband and wife, boyfriend and girlfriend, mother and daughter, and other couples come to see me for the purpose of having a session with each of them. Following a session with a female patient by the name of Ellen, who had a very useful female Spirit Guide, I performed a session on her husband but ran into a brick wall as far as getting his Spirit Guide to come forth. I suspected dark force interference and ended the session abruptly. I decided to see if I could re-hypnotize the couple next to each other and see if Ellen's Spirit Guide could help me release foreign energy from her husband. I explained to the couple that this was experimental and that I didn't know if it would work, but it was worth a try. After making certain that these individuals were comfortable with this approach and privacy was not an issue, I began the dual session. The husband's Spirit Guide would still not come forth, but Ellen's Spirit Guide did, and confirmed my suspicions that dark forces were responsible. I asked Ellen's Spirit Guide to help me remove all entities attached to her husband, and that's exactly what her Guide did. I almost said, "Hot damn!" out loud. I was unbelievably excited but was able to keep my composure as her Spirit Guide helped me complete the removal of all foreign energy from her husband, including the exorcism of many dark force entities. Her Spirit Guide also exposed past life memories that were contributing to his issues and followed up with wise advice for him.

This extraordinary technique worked beautifully for couples that came to me; however, I knew that I needed someone nearby with an easily accessible Spirit Guide to help with the single individual patient when I was unable to get to his Spirit Guide. I found such a person who had been a patient, and she worked out well. The success from these dual hypnosis sessions was mind-boggling. Unfortunately, my assistant lived over seventy miles away and did this out of the kindness of her heart. It was becoming progressively obvious that I needed an assistant who lived reasonably close by and had a Spirit Guide who would consistently come forth when called upon.

Once again I was shown that there are no coincidences, and things always happen for a reason. A patient that I had seen several years ago came for a return visit and has since become a hypnotherapist. She agreed to assist me in these dual hypnosis sessions and has been doing so for several years. Many Spirit Guides are extremely gifted. A very helpful and valid Spirit Guide who consistently comes forth when called upon is really all that's needed when carrying out a dual hypnosis. I have witnessed many such Spirit Guides help me remove foreign energy, zero in on past lifetimes that have caused or contributed to the patient's problem, and then come up with extremely helpful suggestions for the patient.

Following many hundreds of dual hypnosis cases, it became obvious that the dark forces were present 100% of the time in the patients that I was unable to have a Spirit Guide come forth. Also, the majority of these same patients were not able to achieve regression. Therefore, I am able to occasionally regress a patient whose Spirit Guide is being held back by dark forces. I am sure that dark forces, and probably powerful dark forces, are also responsible for preventing the regression of these patients.

Most patients were quite satisfied with the dual hypnosis sessions and they didn't feel that further sessions were necessary, since all foreign energy, and especially the dark forces, were removed and all their issues were addressed and taken care of in a very complete fashion. In addition, they were also taught protective measures which would help protect against future entity infestation. As time went on, these protective measures, namely utilizing God Light visualizations and affirmations, proved to be very effective as did the avoidance of vulnerable situations.

The several dual hypnosis patients that did decide to return for a solo session were elated in that they were now able to successfully call forth a Spirit Guide and be regressed to past lifetimes. An interesting aspect of these repeat solo sessions following a dual session is that these patients had been very good about protecting themselves with the God Light visualization and affirmation and avoidance of vulnerable situations. At the time of the subsequent solo hypnotic session, they had no foreign energy present as reported by their Spirit Guides.

Patients who have a solo session years after a dual session and have not protected themselves properly will almost always have attached entities, especially dark forces, and be once again unable to regress or reach a Spirit Guide. I feel that these patients somehow allow themselves to be more susceptible to entity infestation, especially powerful dark forces or great numbers of dark forces, who are able to pull off these measures. Exemplary cases of dual hypnosis will be presented in Chapter Fourteen.

REMOTE ENTITY RELEASEMENT

Dr. Baldwin also removed entities remotely and coined the term "remote spirit releasement." I was becoming progressively more eager to try this out, so when the opportunity presented itself, I jumped at the chance so I could use the patient's Spirit Guide to accomplish this. The original case in point was a woman who had a daughter who wanted her mother and me to resolve her severe emotional problems.

I decided to have the mother act as an intermediary and have her Spirit Guide locate her daughter and get permission from her daughter's Higher Self to check for and release any foreign energy that was attached to her. Once this permission had been obtained, I carried out a remote entity releasement on the daughter using the mother's Spirit Guide.

This worked quite well; however the success I was observing from the dual hypnosis sessions was so impressive that I decided to utilize my assistant to help with the remote sessions that were requested by people who are not able to come in. These requests for removing entities remotely were either for the people calling or for a loved one who asked them to call. This was a good decision, as I look back on this, for I once again began to hear about unbelievable improvement, but now it was occurring in the people being remotely depossessed. I have completed many hundreds of these cases and have received much in the way of positive feedback.

My assistant's Spirit Guide as well as other Spirit Guides have been of great assistance in helping me carry out dual hypnosis and remote entity releasement sessions. These Spirit Guides not only released entities remotely, they discovered past lives that contributed to the patient's problems and came up with much-needed advice. Once remote entity releasement has been completed, I will ask my assistant's Spirit Guide to send the remote patient love and light, and later I will call and encourage the remote patient to routinely carry out the protective measures. If a family member or friend is used as an intermediary, I will encourage that person to either see that the remote patient consistently utilizes the protective measures or does this for him. Remote entity releasement is discussed in greater detail in Chapter Fifteen.

THE IMPORTANCE OF BEING CREATIVE AND WORKING WITH SPIRIT GUIDES

My purpose in writing this book is to pass on what I have learned so as to expand the vision of conventional medicine. My experience with past life regression therapy tells me that people in their present lifetime are the sum total of all their previous personalities and are very much influenced by past life memories which may surface due to an interaction with a person, place, or event in their present lifetime. My experience also tells me that people may be affected by their future lifetimes and that time does not exist in the spiritual dimension, which means that the past, present, and future are all occurring simultaneously. Throw in past present-life influences and the presence of attached entities or energy beings, and you now have a conglomeration of powerful influences that can change the nature or behavior of a human being. Rarely these changes are positive or inspirational and can promote benevolent behavior or be responsible for one's talent. Unfortunately, most of the resulting effects are detrimental and account for a good many of the physical and emotional problems that people endure. In other words, these influences are one of the main causes of the suffering that mankind is experiencing on a daily basis. Medicine can no longer ignore these influences that I and others have found to be extremely real. The time has come for physicians to open their minds and understand that alleviating suffering is the reason they chose a medical career. In order to zero in on the life-changing effects of these major causes, I will attempt to highlight each of these causes by devoting individual chapters to each of them. I will describe and discuss a multiplicity of cases throughout this book for which names and other identifiable information have been changed so as to ensure the privacy of the subjects. Some of these cases will be more detailed and complete, while others will be described in part so as to emphasize a particular aspect of the case. As my thrust transferred from research to a busy practice, I made a less concentrated effort to follow up on each and every case; therefore there will be some cases for which no long term result has been documented.

I will dedicate the next several chapters to the discovery and release of attached entities that I have encountered and at the same time stress the importance of being creative during the process, especially when dealing with the very devious dark forces. In order to accomplish this in a more understandable way, I will discuss the dark forces first and then get into the rather extensive use of Spirit Guides to monitor and confirm the release of these dark force entities and other attachments. Descriptions of other forms of entity attachments and their methods of releasement will follow.

Chapter 4

THE DARK FORCES

My experience in dealing with dark forces has been quite extensive, and I agree with those who have pioneered in the releasement of spirits that there is a hierarchy of powerful dark forces that issue commands to the underling dark force entities who believe without question that they have no light within them and that light is harmful and could even destroy them. These false beliefs are so instilled into the dark force entities that they have no doubts that if they do not carry out the orders and demands of their hierarchy, they will be punished and possibly destroyed.

THE PRETENDERS

Dark force entities can be extremely deceptive and will often pretend to be a Spirit Guide. With this in mind I always test them by saying, "I am immediately sending you a gift of Light. Will you accept it?" A true Spirit Guide would always accept the gift of Light. If I am dealing with a dark force entity it will either say no or not answer; however, very powerful dark force entities can even lie about this and say yes. I therefore find that I must always rely on my intuitive feelings. If I suspect that there is a dark force pretending to be a Spirit Guide, I will ask more questions, paying particular attention to the tone of voice, words chosen, and attitude. Sooner or later the egotistical dark force will show its true colors.

On occasion I will ask, "Do you believe that Jesus Christ is our Savior?"

Some of the responses that I have received include, "No way, José!" and excessive obscenities such as, "Mother f_____," and so on. I have also heard "Yes," from a powerful dark force who acted very much like a Spirit Guide and even identified several dark force entities who were subsequently removed. I became suspicious of this pretender, mostly because of his attitude, and I called for my volunteer Spirit Guide Abel, who confirmed my suspicions and took over. Once again I reiterate that the powerful dark forces will lie and do whatever it takes to be the great pretender.

Many times when I am unable to get a response and I'm convinced that I am dealing with a dark force, I find myself calling them out, much like the gunfight at the OK Corral. A phrase I often use is, "I know you're in there. Have the guts to talk to me!"

DARK EXPERIENCE

I would now like to give the reader the flavor of what it's like to deal with dark force entities. I saw a middle-aged man as a patient who obviously had many dark force entities present. As soon as he entered into hypnosis, he began writhing all over the couch, giving off occasional growls. I felt that the dark force entities knew they were being sought after. All of a sudden this patient sat up, still deeply in trance, and looked directly at me with his eyelids fluttering and said in a very loud, gruff voice, "Who *are* you?"

I simply answered, "I'm the guy who is going to get rid of you." I then helped the patient to recline and successfully removed those dark forces with the assistance of his Spirit Guide.

Another case I encountered involved a man from Australia. I conducted a successful exorcism and removed several dark force entities from him. He returned the following day with the express purpose of telling me that just before I removed those entities he heard a voice say, "He's getting a cross; he's getting a cross."

Whenever I know I'm dealing with dark forces I get up from my chair and go over to a table and pick up a crucifix that I've had since the 4th grade. This lets the dark forces know where I stand and adds power to the process. It has become obvious that they are watching me and know exactly what I'm doing. I have also on occasion heard comments from the dark forces in regard to the patient such as, "He knows the dark side. I am his teacher." I also get direct threats such as, "You don't want to mess with me."

Upon receiving that last threatening comment, I shot back, "You don't want to mess with St. Michael the Archangel."

One of my earliest and most frustrating cases of attempted intimidation by the dark force entities was a gentleman who went deeply into trance and immediately began growling and snarling and jumping up at me at various intervals from a lying position. When this occurred I would then gently place his head and chest back on the couch. The patient then began to howl with his tongue out, while his head and hands shook convulsively. Laughing in an evil fashion he began to display hideous grimaces as he flapped his tongue with his mouth wide open and continued to growl and assume the position of a powerful beast by flexing his arms and legs and curling his hands into what looked like claws. Nothing I said seemed to make any difference. This bizarre behavior continued for over an hour until I decided to wake the patient up. He had no conscious memory of what had occurred. This individual moved away, and I have been unable to contact him. At that time I was unaware of dual hypnosis sessions and remote entity releasements, but I am sure they would have been extremely helpful. It seems that one of the dark force's main objectives is to induce fear, and I have come to the conclusion that once a person becomes fearful, the dark forces have won. I am in full agreement with Dr. Baldwin about the fact that there is a definite battle going on between the forces of good and evil. In my mind the mission of dark force entities is seduction and destruction. They are responsible for very negative and dark thoughts and will often enhance negative emotions and obstruct good intentions whenever possible. They would very much like to see their host carry out evil deeds of all sorts, including murder and suicide. If a patient is suicidal or had such thoughts, you can guarantee the presence of dark forces.

I have found that vulnerability to any uninvited infestation increases under certain conditions. These conditions include distortion of the conscious mind from excessive alcohol, drugs, intense negative emotions such as rage and anger, and when under general anesthesia. (General anesthesia and its relationship to the Foreign Accent Syndrome will be addressed in Chapter Six.) Life on Earth is not easy, and people are often traumatized to the degree that their soul undergoes fragmentation, and they become incomplete souls and thus exceptionally vulnerable to infestation by these foreign energy entities. (This will be covered in more detail in Chapter Eight, Soul Fragments.) Also, one must not forget that these entities can transfer to another individual through sexual interaction. Once again, I am aligned with Dr. Baldwin's thinking in that I also find the dark forces to be arrogant, disruptive, obscene, and full of hostility. Patients describe them as dark forms or hideous creatures of all sorts.

Once all foreign energy and especially dark force entities have been successfully removed and I have a confirmation from the Spirit Guide that they have gone to the proper destinations, I then ask the Spirit Guide if there is any more foreign energy present within the patient. If I get "No further foreign energy is present," I then lead the patient into a God Light visualization which I spoke of previously. This visualization allows the patient to see, feel, or otherwise imagine the spark of God Light within him, expanding, filling his body, and then surrounding him with a protective shield of God Light. I then have the patient promise to carry out this visualization upon waking, before meals, and before going to sleep. I also give him the affirmation that I mentioned earlier. All of this is a reminder so we will not forget our spiritual heritage, who we are. It also sends the message to uninvited foreign energy, especially dark forces, that we are all part of God and captains of our soul, and no, you are not allowed to enter our space.

HARASSMENT BY THE DARK FORCES

I have had many cases that serve as good examples of harassment by dark force entities. For instance I have found that patients often get lost or are unable to find their way to an appointment with me; sometimes they may develop physical problems that could also prevent them from seeing me. When they eventually show up, I have always discovered dark forces. Dark force entities are without exception the bad guys. They know that the patient is seeing me for the purpose of getting rid of them, and they don't like it. They will continue to harass the patient by making him develop a headache, an episode of nausea, a choking sensation, or a pain in various parts of the body during the hypnotic induction. I have always been able to put an immediate end to these symptoms by touching the part of the body involved with a crucifix. Occasionally the patient will sense something pulling on his arm or leg while under hypnosis. Again, touching that arm or leg with a crucifix has, in my experience, always caused the patient to feel an instant release of that extremity.

I have had several cases that bring to mind an unusual phenomenon that I cannot explain; however, I feel very strongly that it is also part of dark force harassment, the purpose of which is to keep the therapist from removing dark forces. In most of these cases, the patient can see his Spirit Guide but is unable to hear him; also the Spirit Guide is sometimes unable to speak through the patient. I have seen this situation multiple times, often with different scenarios, and have found that creativity on the part of the therapist is vital. I have experienced these situations and have been able to successfully carry out the removal of attached entities by eliciting *yes* and *no* answers from the Spirit Guide. The patient is able to see enough of his Guide so as to pass his answers on to the therapist. Thus, methods such as nodding of the Guide's head or raising one or two hands for yes and no would work well. I have also had cases whereupon the Guide was holding the patient's hand, and we would ask the Spirit Guide to squeeze the patient's hand once for *yes*, and twice for *no*. A memorable case involved a patient's Spirit Guide who appeared only as a beam of light and could not speak. I asked if the Guide would allow his light to get brighter for *yes* and dimmer for *no*. It worked.

Another form of harassment is often seen on certain parcels of land where a massacre occurred. Such locations literally bear the stench of evil, and as such, dark forces consider these sites to be their space and thus will bring all sorts of harassment to people who attempt to live there.

CURSES

A curse, hex, or spell is projected negative energy which is cast upon a person by an individual who has a heartfelt wish to bring harm upon that person. It is most likely to come from someone who is involved with voodoo, witchcraft, black magic, or a satanic cult and their rituals. Sometimes the negative emotions that occur during the casting of such spells are so extreme that the soul of the person performing this ritual fragments, and his soul fragment is projected into the victim of the curse, which, according to these demonic people, adds power to the curse and gives them power over the victim. The victims of such rituals are always loaded with dark force and powerful dark force attachments, or Earthbound spirits with excessive dark force attachments, all of whom are charged with the duty to maintain and continue the curse. If the individual made a pact with the dark forces in a past life, he may even have legions of dark forces within him.

ozᒪ⌐Ꙅ૭૭

The exorcisms that I have conducted incorporate some of Dr. Baldwin's techniques, but now they are being put into effect with Spirit Guide confirmation every step of the way. The Spirit Guide's ability to pick up on the frequencies of various entities is unbeliev-ably helpful; moreover, their innate spiritual knowledge that enables them to determine whether entities have been taken to and have arrived at the designated destination is crucial to the process. I will be describing the situations that occur while performing exorcisms, and they in no way compare to what Hollywood has been present-ing to the public. Such movies depicting exorcisms are designed and made to scare the hell out of the audience; the more shocking, the better: people floating, demons appearing, and people screaming and being injured. Entities are real. Dark forces are real. But what is also real is that every human being has that very special spark of its Creator, which makes that person's soul an eternal being which cannot be destroyed.

In *Healing Lost Souls*, Dr. William Baldwin stated that researchers in this field have estimated that 50 to 100% of people will have expe-rienced the effect of entities attached to them at some time in their lives. My experience has revealed that a good 80% of my patients have had entities attached to them. I would very much like to emphasize that these statistics have shown that there is a need to carry out exor-cisms of dark forces and complete removal of all attached entities for a good percent of people living on this Earth. There is also a need to teach people the preventive measures they need to take to remain free of foreign energy and therefore free of excessive problems. The Comprehensive Hypnoregression Therapy protocol I have designed after years of experience practically guarantees complete removal of all attached entities and deals with problems stemming from past lifetimes. I am able to accomplish a lot in one session using a valid and experienced Spirit Guide that has come forth. If dark forces are preventing the Guide from coming through, waking the patient up, or keeping the patient from undergoing hypnosis, a dual hypnosis will accomplish what's needed, even if the patient won't allow himself to be hypnotized. Thus a patient can usually expect good results in one session, but if dark forces are keeping us from accomplishing this, the patient can know up front that a second session utilizing dual hypnosis will for sure achieve the desired result by removing all foreign energy and enabling the patient to confront, understand, and release the negative effects of emotional past life memories.

Chapter 5

POWERFUL DARK FORCES

DEMONS CAN BE DRAMATIC

A case that involved a middle-aged female fashion designer from California was one that caused an exceptionally tense atmosphere to exist throughout the session. This woman came to me with an array of problems including eye pain, diagnosed as ocular hypertension, scratchy throat and cough that makes clearing her throat almost impossible, being consumed with darkness and negativity, and giving up easily when it comes to overcoming obstacles. I suspected the presence of dark forces when I was unable to regress her or get to her Spirit Guide. The same situation occurred during a follow up session, but when I forcefully said to the patient under hypnosis that I needed her Spirit Guide to come forward, I heard the patient say, "No." I then said that I would like the one who answered to please tell me what your purpose is. The answer I received was, "Darkness, and to live."

The patient came to see me during the years when I first began using an assistant to conduct dual hypnosis sessions. This assistant, who lived seventy miles away, had a Spirit Guide that proved to be exceptionally good and very helpful. As I look back on this case I can honestly say that I was not totally prepared for what was to come. The dual hypnosis session began with my assistant's Spirit Guide revealing a large number of Earthbound spirits and extraterrestrials, which were contributing to the patient's problems. When I asked my assistant's Spirit Guide about dark forces, I was told that they numbered in the many hundreds and included one very powerful dark force entity. I immediately took my crucifix in hand and initiated the exorcism utilizing extra help from St. Michael the Archangel and another great warrior Archangel, Metatron. The battle continued for over a half hour, when I was told that six dark force entities won't leave. I then called in the rest of the Archangels, as many Master Spirits as I could find, and St. Germain, to help. After fifteen minutes the Spirit Guide said that all the dark forces have been encapsulated, and that St. Michael the Archangel has taken them to the Light. Sighing a breath of relief, I now turned my attention to the remaining extraterrestrials and Earthbound spirits. Following an interrogation and an understanding of their relationship to the patient, they were removed. The last Earthbound spirit interviewed would not initially speak, but with enough prodding he finally admitted that he was responsible for all the patient's negative emotions, including blackness. The Spirit Guide immediately identified him as the powerful dark force entity who had pretended to be an Earthbound spirit. I quickly re-invoked the presence of special angels and the two Archangels St. Michael and Metatron. As the battle ensued, I noticed that my assistant's face contorted in a fearful manner as her Spirit Guide cried out, "The powerful dark force has talons around the patient's throat!"

At that very moment the patient began to gag and cough. I called for more reinforcements as the Spirit Guide said, "This is a delicate procedure." The patient stopped coughing, and I was told that the powerful dark force had been taken away by St. Michael the Archangel.

I now called for the patient's Spirit Guide to come forth, asking, "Will you help?"

I heard, "Yes." But further questions yielded no answers.

I then asked my assistant's Spirit Guide, "Why am I receiving no answers to my questions?"

My assistant's Spirit Guide then replied that she sees a male figure next to the patient. I again asked more questions and pressed for more information from this Spirit, who was acting as the patient's Spirit Guide but was no longer communicating. As I did, the patient once again began to cough and choke. My assistant's Spirit Guide cried out, "The male figure has turned dark, and again I am seeing talons around the patient's neck. This is the same powerful dark force entity that was taken away. He did something only a powerful dark force could do; he split, and only part of him was taken away, and part of him remained."

Shaking off the feeling of utter astonishment I hurriedly began a third exorcism and with a sense of urgency asked the Archangels St. Michael and Metatron how best we could remove this entity. I was told, "The patient needs to know how the presence of this entity has served her."

I then asked the patient to forgive herself for going along with the darkness. After complying with this request the patient told me that she felt less pressure on her throat, but within a few seconds she began to cry and screamed, "I can't see the spark of God Light within me... it's gone!"

I solicited more power from the two Archangels, and as I did, my assistant's Spirit Guide spoke to the patient, saying, "Whatever dark thing you have participated in, and you don't even have to know the story–just encapsulate it in light, and be willing to let it go. A powerful dark force entity can even hide your light and keep you from seeing it."

At this time I decided to call in the remaining Archangels, powerful Master Spirits, many more Rescue Spirits of Light, and finally I asked for help from Jesus. Within a few minutes my assistant's Spirit Guide said, "Jesus is here, and so are all else who have been called. I cannot do any more; it is up to the patient." At that moment I told the patient to really focus and imagine, feel, sense, and see the spark of God Light within her. A few moments later the patient became calm and peaceful as the Spirit Guide spoke the words, "The powerful dark force has been carried away by St. Michael the Archangel."

I then led the patient through the God Light visualization and affirmation and thought to myself, "Chalk up one more for the power of good."

Several weeks later the patient informed me that she had markedly improved in her symptoms, namely feeling lighter, with no further eye pain and having less coughing with the ability to clear her throat right away. She also said she is no longer consumed with darkness and now has an aversion to negativity and negative emotions, which makes her feel younger and gives her a great attitude with the ability to overcome most obstacles.

Since the experience of the late Dr. Baldwin has also become my experience, I now began to routinely inquire about the presence of powerful dark force entities instead of waiting for the Spirit Guide to inform me that one is present.

This was one of my earliest cases of entity releasement. As I gained experience I learned to ask about and remove dark forces, and especially powerful dark forces first, so as not to give powerful dark forces the option of hiding, and I hadn't yet discovered the effectiveness of using the crucifix to negate the effect of the dark forces on various parts of the patient's body.

SPIRIT GUIDES CAN PANIC, TOO

This young woman from Canada came to see me because of a constant feeling of anxiety which has remained for many years. She confessed that as a teenager she was involved in witchcraft activities which took place in a certain room in a house that her family had moved into when she was ten years old. Occasionally she would sense the presence of a strange man in that room, which sometimes made her feel paralyzed. Her family and friends experienced the same feelings when they were in that room. Also, her adolescent niece came to live in that house at a later time and began practicing witchcraft in that same room. The patient moved out in her late teens and then moved back home for a few years. It was at that time that her anxiety began.

Under deep hypnosis I had the patient call for her Spirit Guide. The answers we received came from an entity, not the Spirit Guide. When I asked the entity what its purpose was in being here, he blurted out, "I want to be with her... I love her!" Asking more questions, it soon became obvious that this entity never had a human body and was dark. Further discussion with this entity revealed the presence of many more dark forces. I explained that as a dark force entity, he should not feel love, and used this to my advantage by asking questions regarding what the dark forces had told him, namely that he had no spark of Light within him and that light is harmful. I then asked him to look deeply within the center of his very being for a spark of Light.

The dark force kept denying that he had such a spark of Light within him; however I kept prodding him on to find it, which he finally did. I then asked, "How does it make you feel when you look at it?"

He responded, "Happy."

"But you're not supposed to be happy." I continued on with this back and forth banter but soon discovered that the dark force was going to need an exorcism, which I then began. During the exorcism the dark force entity notified me that he absolutely refused to be encapsulated in a capsule of Light. I quickly informed him that this capsule of Light would protect him from being dragged away by other dark force entities to be punished for even considering the presence of light within him. The dark force remained resistant to the encapsulation until I finally said, "Once you are in the Light you will be permanently protected from punishment by the dark force hierarchy, and you can also love this individual from the Light."

Finally the encapsulation of the dark force was accomplished, and he was then taken to the special place in the Light by St. Michael the

Archangel, where he definitely chose to enter the Light. I was now able to communicate with the patient's Spirit Guide, who told me that the patient still had legions of dark force entities attached to her. Once again I set up a perimeter defense with warrior angels of Light and Legions of Heaven and called for the Rescue Spirits of Light to encapsulate all dark force entities. The battle was long and arduous, and twenty minutes into it the Spirit Guide cried out in a panicky voice, "There's too many of them!" I then called for more Rescue Spirits of Light and other reinforcements, which finally turned the tide. After a total of forty minutes, all but one of the dark forces had been encapsulated in Light. The remaining dark force was described by the Spirit Guide as a very powerful dark force, who was exceptionally adept at hiding. By this time I had already invoked the help of St. Michael the Archangel to take away the encapsulated dark forces. I now asked St. Michael the Archangel to also help with the encapsulation of this powerful one. Fifteen minutes later the powerful dark force was encapsulated and also taken away by St. Michael the Archangel. The patient's Spirit Guide now in a relaxed voice exclaimed that all dark force entities have been taken away. We then turned our attention to the removal of several Earthbound souls and followed with a God Light visualization and affirmation.

POWERFUL PRETENDERS ALSO PLAY HIDE AND SEEK

I have had many cases involving powerful dark forces that required reinforcements to accomplish their proper removal. These dark forces elude capture and will fight tooth and toenail to avoid Light encapsulation. On several occasions I have witnessed a patient's apprehensive and fearful expression during the time that a spiritual battle is occurring in an attempt to encapsulate a powerful dark force. If I see that facial expression change dramatically to a smug, defiant look, often accompanied by uncontrollable, evil laughter, I know that the powerful dark force is reacting through the patient and feeling triumphant, and it's time to call in reinforcements.

This case brings out the fact that powerful dark forces will lie about anything. Testing Spirit Guides is all well and good, but when powerful dark forces are involved, all bets are off, and the therapist has to rely on his Higher Self and his intuition to figure things out.

Sarah was a 26-year-old patient that was brought to me by her husband. Sarah had been diagnosed as having a manic depressive condition and has remained exceptionally moody. She had seen physicians in their home town in Colorado, but to no avail.

Sarah easily entered deep hypnosis, and when she called for a Spirit Guide, an answer came through from Titus, who accepted a gift of Light; however his manner of speaking made me uncomfortable, so I decided to summon Abel, my volunteer Spirit Guide. Abel arrived and we removed dark forces and soul fragments. While I was having Sarah work through a God Light visualization, Abel interrupted and said, "I see a dark opening in the God Light. It is a very powerful dark force who has been hiding." Abel then exclaimed in a loud voice, "It's Titus!" I called the warrior angels of Light and Legions of Heaven to set up a perimeter defense and then called in the Rescue Spirits of Light and all the reinforcements, namely all the Archangels, and as many Master Spirits as I could gather. The battle took a little while but soon the powerful dark force was subdued within a Light capsule and taken to the Light.

In a follow up call several weeks later I was told by Sarah's husband that she became worse for a few days following the session and then felt great.

MASTERS OF OBSTRUCTION

Margaret was a 35-year-old woman from British Columbia who had an intense desire to help people and also had all the signs of being a Light Worker. A Light Worker is a person with an exceptional amount of God Light who is motivated to do good work which makes the world a better place, improves peoples' lives, and/or elevates people to a higher level of consciousness. At the same time, she also exhibited signs of being held back and controlled by an exceptionally evil force. She had lost the desire to do things that she loved and found that she was no longer able to meditate, which resulted in varying degrees of depression. Margaret intuitively knew that she had psychic gifts and was able to channel her Spirit Guide. She also had been told by psychics that she had lifetimes in, and therefore a direct connection to Lemuria, ancient Egypt, India, Africa, Greece, and Persia. During a massage she experienced a vision whereupon she was visited by an extraterrestrial who told her that she will be lecturing and carrying out spiritual teaching; however, at the same time she was very aware that she has had stage fright since she was a child. She has had lucid dreams where she has seen herself attempting to help people and then being burned to death as a witch. She also somehow felt that she was responsible for people dying as a result of her attempting to help them.

Margaret went to a hypnotherapist for past life regression but was blocked from seeing anything except for a very evil-looking Reptilian eye. The therapist began to choke and cough and could not continue the session. He later told Margaret that he felt he was being attacked. When Margaret tried to help a good friend not have suicidal feelings, Margaret herself began to have a coughing frenzy. Later she found that she would affect coworkers and people around her to the point where they would become negative and uncomfortable.

I began the hypnotic session and almost at once was in contact with Margaret's Spirit Guide, who identified six dark forces, some of whom were powerful. I immediately started the exorcism procedure but soon found that Margaret's Spirit Guide was quite frustrated. There seemed to be an obstruction to any progress that was being made. At this moment Margaret's Spirit Guide said, "Someone is laughing at you and blocking me from seeing anything." Feeling the Spirit Guide's frustration, I decided to ask the Spirit Guide when these dark forces entered this lifetime. The Guide said, "They entered as a young child; they pretended to be good and in need of help, so she felt sorry for them and accepted them so she could help them."

One hour had passed with no progress in removing the dark forces; but hearing what Margaret's Spirit Guide had to say struck my mind like a bolt of lightning. I immediately told Margaret that these dark forces had taken advantage of her young mind and her strong desire to help others. I also felt that these dark forces had performed similar feats on her in past lifetimes and that these actions have haunted her because she has experienced much guilt about people dying because of her actions. I raised my voice and made it very clear to Margaret that she needs to forgive herself for allowing dark forces to enter her in this lifetime as well as in past lifetimes. I then said this forgiveness needs to be genuine and come from the heart. Margaret had been crying throughout this ordeal but now it became accelerated and then came to a complete halt as she spoke the words, "I forgive myself."

At that moment the obstruction faded, and the Spirit Guide could now see what was happening and said, "The dark forces have left on their own."

I then asked the Spirit Guide about Earthbound spirits and was told, "Margaret is too strong for Earthbound spirits to attach; however, she does have several extraterrestrials hovering over her. They are benevolent extraterrestrials from Pleiades who are here to protect her. They tell me that when Margaret first became pregnant, the Reptilians attacked and converted her normal pregnancy into an ectopic pregnancy which required surgery. The Reptilians do not want her to reproduce and bring more Light Workers into this world."

Margaret's Spirit Guide and I agreed to leave the benevolent extraterrestrials so they would be able to help Margaret. Margaret's soul was found to be complete, so I followed with powerful suggestions and instructions on protection so as to prevent further infestation by dark forces or demonic Reptilians.

THE POWERFUL DARK FORCE ENTITY WHO KNOWS ME

Judith Baldwin, Dr. William Baldwin's widow, told me that as Dr. Baldwin continued to remove dark force entities he began to run into more powerful dark forces. I have had that experience as well; also my work is definitely getting the attention of the dark forces and their powerful hierarchy. I say this because during the past several years the powerful dark forces have found it necessary to bring me messages through my patients. One such patient was a woman by the name of Rebecca, who was inundated with dark thoughts. A friend of hers who was a psychic told her that she was possessed by something dark. Being unsuccessful at connecting with Rebecca's Spirit Guide under deep hypnosis, I found myself communicating with an entity by the name of Seth.

Rebecca was extremely nervous and felt that something did not want her to proceed with what we were doing. I was told by Seth that Rebecca was infested with dark forces. I thought that Seth was an Earthbound spirit who was offering his help, but I wasn't sure, so I began to interrogate him further. His answers to my questions were appropriate until I asked him about his purpose in being here. His answer was one I have heard several times before. He said, "I love to do this." It was now obvious to me that I was dealing with a dark force who was most likely a powerful dark force. I once again called for a Spirit Guide. Rebecca felt a presence and could see a figure encased by bright light who identified himself as a Spirit Guide and accepted a gift of Light. I had a good feeling about the validity of this Spirit Guide, who then confirmed the presence of legions of dark force entities and identified Seth as a powerful dark force.

The patient now exhibited a great many facial grimaces and began speaking unintelligible gibberish as her body moved in strange ways. All the Archangels and several Master Spirits were necessary to carry out the exorcism. The battle continued for over thirty minutes, when Rebecca's Spirit Guide blurted out that all dark force entities had been removed; however, Seth had been rescued by the dark forces. Once again I was hearing something I had heard before, and I thought to myself, "It figures. He's a powerful dark force."

At this moment Rebecca took on the persona of an evil entity and exhibited an evil smile. Her Spirit Guide yelled out that another powerful dark force had appeared, and this one was extremely powerful in the hierarchy of the dark forces. The patient now rolled her head towards me, still under deep hypnosis, as the powerful dark force began to speak through Rebecca. It said, "You know me... we go back a long way." According to the Spirit Guide, the powerful dark force entity then left. I followed with the usual suggestions for God Light protection and then ended the session with many questions in my mind.

Several weeks later I saw a 12-year-old girl who had several dark force entities present. Using her Spirit Guide, we completed the exorcism. I then asked her Guide if all dark force entities had been removed by St. Michael the Archangel. The answer I received from her Spirit Guide was, "All but one, and he has a message for you." The message was, "You know me... we will talk again." I then asked the patient's Spirit Guide to tell me who was speaking to me. Her Guide replied, "This is a very powerful dark force entity."

I responded, "Please call for St. Michael the Archangel and ask him what is going on with this powerful dark force who knows me."

St. Michael the Archangel then told me, through the 12-year-old patient, that this powerful dark force was the French nobleman whom I had befriended when I was a French knight centuries ago. He became quite evil, grabbing off power any way he could, thus causing the relationship to deteriorate. St. Michael the Archangel then followed with "You were aware of his evil deeds at that time and therefore broke off your friendship with him. He is very high in the hierarchy of the dark forces."

I have since confirmed what St. Michael the Archangel told me about this powerful dark force with Abel, the volunteer Spirit Guide, Master Spirits, and from my former patient, Evelyn, who was my half-sister in that medieval life. Evidently this powerful dark force has lived in a human body. Truly this information appears to contradict what Dr. Baldwin said about dark forces, namely that they are non-human and have never lived in a human body. Once again I will repeat we will never know exactly how the spirit world works until we are there in spirit form. A third communication occurred several months later when another patient's Spirit Guide said a powerful dark force was saying, "You know me... I will see you again."

One year later my wife and I were witness to a paranormal event that bore the stench of evil. We decided to sit outside on the patio before retiring for the night. It was a clear night except for two or three clouds above us. We conversed for several minutes until I inadvertently looked up at the sky again and told my wife to do the same. What we saw happening was mind-blowing. The few small clouds that I observed earlier were now breaking up into smaller clouds, moving in different directions and taking on various configurations that seemed to be joining together and separating, as if to form a pattern against the night sky. Within a matter of minutes it became obvious that we were both looking at what appeared to be a devil's face. Two rounded rectangular shaped clouds of the same size had formed the eyes, and two rounded clouds, the ears, as two opposing half-moon shaped clouds fell into place, looking very much like horns. An elongated cloud at the bottom of the formation then took on the shape of a sinister sneer. We both agreed that this was not our imagination. The clouds that formed the ears, eyes, and horns, were perfectly symmetrical in size and shape. While our attention was riveted to this ominous scene in the night sky, I looked at my wife and said, "Yep! Another message." The pattern that had formed began to break up within minutes.

Approximately ten months later I received a fifth message, once again through a patient. This particular patient had an extensive list of problems, including anxiety, depression, claustrophobia, and many fears. I had seen him previously and removed many entities, including several powerful dark forces. Many dark forces were once again removed during his present session, which was about to be completed when his Spirit Guide yelled out, "There is a powerful dark force here, and he is saying, 'Kill yourself.'"

I immediately asked his Spirit Guide, "Who is he speaking to?"

The Spirit Guide answered, "You! Now he's telling me that he knows you and that he will be coming for you."

I answered this powerful dark force by telling him, "I send you Light and love from Jesus, all the Archangels, all the Master Spirits and St. Germain," and followed with, "I will continue to help people and be on the side of good, and yes, we will overcome evil."

Rather than end this true but dark story on a dark note, I would also like to mention that I have been routinely asking St. Michael the Archangel to help me with patients prior to seeing each patient. A short while after I made this decision and was faithfully carrying it out, I had what I feel was another paranormal experience, but this time it was a good one. While going through my usual routine to get to my e-mail and finally clicking the mouse on "E-mail," I was amazed but at the same time very gratified to see a large picture of St. Michael the Archangel appear on my computer screen. This picture had been placed on an icon that I did not even get near. In my mind, this was also a message–a good one.

It seems to me that the dark forces and especially the powerful dark forces are exceptionally real, and once again I was shown how real. Some time ago I became curious to see if it was possible to pick up sounds that were not perceptible to the human ear during an exorcism. I have been able to communicate with dark force entities as well as other entities through my patients while they are in the theta brainwave frequency, which is predominantly present during the hypnotic altered state of consciousness; however, I could hear nothing in the way of extraneous noise or speaking during the actual exorcism. My experience tells me that the dark forces don't go quietly, so I feel very strongly that human ears are not able to pick up these voices and noises, and I attribute this lack of audible sound to the fact that dark forces exist in another dimension, and the sounds made during an exorcism most likely occur in a different frequency that is not perceptible to the human ear.

With the patient's permission, I recorded a session whereupon I removed a large number of dark forces and powerful dark forces and sent it to a recording expert who used special software and headphones to see if he could pick up sounds not heard by myself or my patient during that session. As it turns out, he reported hearing noises such as snaps, clicks, and panicky whispering, and the name "Michael" growled in a demonic voice. I would like to remind the reader that St. Michael the Archangel plays a major role in the exorcism by removing the dark forces after they are encapsulated.

I obviously have gotten the attention of the dark forces, and yes, they're getting personal with me. They don't like what I am doing, especially the fact that I found a way to get around their keeping me from regressing the patient or having the patient's Spirit Guide come forward. Thus the technique of using another person's Spirit Guide in a dual hypnosis session has enabled me to overcome their dark obstruction and has allowed me to carry out a successful exorcism with Spirit Guide confirmation and a removal of all foreign energy from patients.

Well, I still feel that things happen for a reason, and somehow I have discovered a path that I feel compelled to follow. Using Comprehensive Hypnoregression Therapy, I have been able to put an end to the suffering that many people endure because conventional medicine has not yet considered such therapy. The sheer volume of positive feedback that I have received from my patients has inspired and motivated me to write this book and share what I have learned. My goal is to have conventional medicine take notice and begin to understand the importance of such therapy. In doing so, I will be helping the power of good defeat the power of evil, and no, I won't be intimidated.

Chapter 6

EARTHBOUND SPIRITS

I would now like to shed light on the most common entity attachment, the Earthbound spirit. This is the soul of a deceased human being, also known as a disembodied human spirit, and the consciousness that survives following a person's death. This soul declines going to the Light for many reasons, such as confusion (not realizing he has died); a mother wanting to watch over her children; or continued cravings, such as with drug addiction, to name a few. These Earthbound spirits remain in the so called lower astral plane, where some of them decide to attach to living human beings for many reasons. Most of these reasons are self-serving, and some are for the benefit of the patient/host. According to Dr. Baldwin, these entities can be enmeshed in the aura, the energy field that surrounds the body, or they may attach to one of the chakras. In simple terms, chakras are considered the "force centers" or invisible whorls of energy located at various points within the physical body that receive and transmit life-force energy. The Earthbound spirit can also attach on or inside the body of the host.

On many occasions I have found that there is not only a difference in the thinking and the wishes of the Earthbound spirit and the patient/host, but rather a clash that results in the patient actually arguing with himself. One can easily see that the personality of the

Earthbound spirit, with all its attributes, detriments, likes and dislikes, can easily interfere with those of the host; however, the most important effect that the Earthbound spirit can have upon its unsuspecting host is that the physical ailments, emotional problems, and addictive tendencies that were present in the Earthbound spirit's lifetime will now be imprinted upon the mind and body of the host. Thus, if the Earthbound spirit had a peptic ulcer and was depressed in his lifetime, the host will most likely develop these conditions. If a person is very near the scene of a fatal accident or in a hospital when someone dies, the proximity to such a death puts the patient/host in a very vulnerable situation. The Earthbound spirit of the deceased may find himself in a confused state, not realizing he has died, and immediately attach to the patient/host who is in the vicinity. As long as we are speaking about increased vulnerability, I would like to say that most people have no clue about how vulnerable they can become while under anesthesia. Millions of major and minor surgeries are performed each year in hospitals and clinics all over the world. This is definitely a frequent and common way for people to open themselves up to entity infestation. Physicians and dentists use various forms of sedation and anesthesia for their procedures, and the public is only too happy to be "out of it" during the procedure. On rare occasions a patient wakes up with a rather bizarre and unpredictable side effect of the procedure, namely speaking with an unusual foreign accent. The medical profession calls this the "foreign accent syndrome," a rare disorder, so rare that only sixty-plus cases have been documented throughout the world since the early 1900s. This so-called syndrome is thought to be somehow associated with various areas of brain injury. The variety of foreign accents that have occurred in people who normally spoke Americanized English language includes Italian, Spanish, German, Russian, Chinese, Jamaican, and Swedish. It may very well be that a tiny brain injury is the culprit; however, I would love to hypnotize some of these people and rule out an entity attachment.

These Earthbound spirits, when attached, are in reality parasitic infestations, as are all attachments, and as such are continually drawing energy from their host, regardless of their reasons for attaching. Some Earthbound spirits may join their host with very sincere intentions of helping him with his Earthly problems, and they may truly be helpful. This often poses a problem for the patient in regard to the releasement of these entities. According to several Master Spirits, Earthbound spirits often search for a host who is kind and has a temperament and personality similar to theirs.

Earthbound spirits may also have attachments. If the Earthbound spirit has a dark force entity attached to him, he and the patient will both be affected by this dark, destructive influence. This Earthbound spirit can now become very hostile, especially in regard to leaving the patient and going to the Light. It is essential to remove the dark force entities that have attached to the Earthbound spirit before attempting to get the Earthbound spirit to voluntarily go to the Light.

Earthbound spirits retain much of their human qualities, and as such I just have to tell you about instances of 'snitching' that I have run in to, when a patient has several Earthbound attachments. I will usually interview each Earthbound spirit and ask if he or she had the patient's particular problem during his or her lifetime. For instance, I would ask, "Did you experience chronic anxiety when you were alive?"

On several occasions I would get answers such as, "No... but so-and-so did," then naming another Earthbound soul who was also attached to that same patient. A group of Earthbound spirits who are attached to an individual seems to resemble a family, with knowledge of each other's weaknesses and secrets, and they are not adverse to engaging in gossip.

I find it amazing that so many of the unusual conditions and problems that befall people today are due to the influence of these Earthbound souls that are attached. Many cases come to mind. One man was so claustrophobic he refused to drive in traffic and often considered two or three people near him to be a crowd, and therefore something to be avoided. He believed that these situations, plus others, were hemming him in, causing him to feel smothered. Once the Earthbound spirit who was the cause of his problem was discovered and sent to the Light, the patient no longer felt that these situations were a problem and intentionally worked his way into crowds and chose to drive in traffic so as to dare the anxiety to return. It didn't. I've had other patients conduct themselves in the same way so as to prove to themselves that they are really cured.

Currently there is a great interest in the subject of being gay. I have had several patients who are homosexual, and most of them had Earthbound spirits who were either homosexual in their lifetimes or members of the opposite sex, who attached when their host was extremely young. I ran across an example of this when I saw two sisters from Australia, both of whom had homosexual tendencies all their adolescent and adult lives. I discovered an Earthbound spirit on each of them, who had joined them in early childhood. The older sister's Earthbound spirit was a male who died in his twenties and said that his purpose for joining was to have fun through her. The younger sister's Earthbound spirit was in his early thirties when he died and said his purpose was to have fun by being her. I often wonder whose personality became dominant as these patients grew up.

I have seen several patients who were writers who came to me because they felt that there was a blockage, something holding them back and preventing them from writing in a creative fashion. Some of these patients were men, and some were women, and all of them were genuinely concerned about this obstruction in their professional life. Some of the blockages were due to past life situations, however others were clearly caused by the influence of Earthbound spirits. When I discover a large number of Earthbound spirits attached to a patient with this problem, I would ask if there are any authors present among the Earthbound spirits, and if so, please step forward. I would then interview this Earthbound spirit and uncover as much information as I could so as to solve the patient's problem. I've often wondered if famous people who die ever decline going to the Light and eventually attach to an individual as an Earthbound spirit.

Well, my answer came quickly during a session with a gentleman writer from North Carolina. Following my request to step forward, a famous author from the 1800s did just that and was very helpful in solving the patient's problem.

Chapter Twelve contains confirmatory information on this subject, which I received from the spiritual mentor of a patient who was Edgar Cayce. I was told that the soul of a famous person usually declines going to the Light following death, after which he may search for–and attach to–a host whom he feels is somewhat talented and has the potential to complete this famous Earthbound spirit's unfinished business. Sometimes such an arrangement can be very successful, but when it is not, it may cause an obstruction to what the host is attempting to accomplish.

Emotional quirks or reactions of an Earthbound spirit can easily affect a host's reactions to environmental situations. Much of what occurs depends upon the degree of possession. I have seen several cases where the Earthbound spirit of a miscarried fetus affects the patient to a greater extent due to the depth of its connection to the human host who was to be its mother. The spirit of these tiny fetuses may be responsible for unusual reactions such as fear, which is reflected in the mother's voice or body language and is not proportionate or appropriate to the situation in which she finds herself. I have also come upon the soul of a dead fetal twin who attached to its twin while still growing in the mother's uterus.

The rate of success in curing patients of a problem that is related to the presence of these tiny Earthbound spirits is phenomenal and therefore very similar to the general success rate seen when entities responsible for the patient's problems are removed. Once Earthbound spirits are sent to the Light they are gone and have no further effect on the patient.

Whenever I touch upon the subject of miscarriages I feel a great sadness come over me. The memories of bringing thousands of healthy babies into the world gave me great joy, which unfortunately was diluted with the unmitigated sadness I experienced while caring for patients having a miscarriage or stillbirth. On many occasions the very early and extremely tiny fetus would come out of the mother moving its arms and legs and having facial grimaces. Seeing this miniature infant moving in this way and feeling his body move as I handed him off to the nurse only added to the atmosphere of gloom that hovered over me and filled the delivery room. This very small fetus was not ready for life outside his mother's womb. He would die shortly, and we all knew it. Many times the mother was awake and crying hysterically. Through the many years of practice I attempted to disconnect myself emotionally from these very sad moments in peoples' lives. It didn't happen; I always felt their pain.

THE TENACIOUS EARTHBOUND SPIRIT

The following case represents a sterling example of an Earthbound spirit attaching to a human being many years ago, detaching when that person died, and reattaching to that same person in a present lifetime. This case also poses a troubling question for which we have no answer. I would like you, the reader, to pay close attention to the details, keeping in mind that 'time' is a construct of the physical world and is not present in the spiritual dimension. This means the past, present, and future are all taking place simultaneously.

A woman in her early thirties from North Dakota, whom I shall refer to as Beverly was brought in to see me by her husband. She had a serious alcohol addiction, and her husband was running out of patience. During the hypnotic session I had the patient call for her Spirit Guide but had no response. I then said, "Is anyone in there besides Beverly?" I heard an affirmative reply and then asked, "Are you Beverly's Spirit Guide?" Again I heard no response. I then asked, "Were you ever in your own human body?" I heard a yes the second time and decided to interview this Earthbound spirit. I started out by asking, "Did you drink alcohol heavily in your lifetime?"

"Yes."

"Did you die of a disease?"

"Yes."

"An alcohol related disease?"

"Yes, liver cirrhosis."

"What is your name?"

"Adam."

I continued the interview; however, I was almost certain that this Earthbound spirit by the name of Adam was the source of the patient's addiction. Since I still didn't have a Spirit Guide on board, I decided to be creative and asked Adam, the Earthbound spirit, to call for *his* Spirit Guide. It worked, as Adam's female Spirit Guide answered, "I am here." Adam's Spirit Guide accepted my gift of Light and was willing to help me. I then asked Adam if he would like to continue his spiritual journey and go to the Light, and if he did, I would be glad to help him do so. Adam agreed, and I wished him Godspeed as he entered the Light. His Spirit Guide was very accommodating, and after confirming Adam's ascent to the Light she helped me remove all foreign energy from the patient.

I later took the patient back to a life that she shared with her present husband, if such a life existed. She went back to a life in the 1920s and recognized her husband as her boyfriend in that lifetime. Her name in that life was Alice, and her boyfriend's name was Gregory. It soon became evident that Alice had a serious alcohol addiction in that life as well. Alice's drinking caused Gregory much pain, so much so that he decided to leave her permanently. Out of intuitive curiosity I wondered if Adam, the alcoholic-inducing Earthbound spirit, was also attached to the patient in that lifetime. I just had to ask, so I said, "Adam, are you attached to Alice?"

Once again I heard, "Yes." After asking more questions it became obvious that Adam, the Earthbound spirit who had an alcohol addiction and had died of this in a past lifetime, was also attached to Alice in this life as well. Adam's Spirit Guide came forward as she did in the previous session. I attempted to remove Adam once again but soon found that he was extremely belligerent and refused to go to the Light. Suspecting that dark forces were attached to Adam and confirming this with his Spirit Guide, I then carried out an exorcism with Adam's Spirit Guide's help and removed several dark force entities from Adam, who now became much more amenable to going to the Light, which he did. With Adam no longer attached to Alice, she underwent an unbelievable change in that lifetime and became completely free from alcohol. Alice and Gregory reunited and soon married and were extremely happy throughout that lifetime.

Now, I have a question for you: would that lifetime in the 1920s have turned out differently if Adam, the alcohol-addicted attachment, had been allowed to remain with Alice? Remember, past, present and future events are theoretically happening simultaneously. By removing entities in that past lifetime, we may have changed past events and re-scripted that lifetime, thus altering history. You decide.

By the way, my patient Beverly spoke to me over a month later and said that she has had no further desire for alcohol and has been completely alcohol-free. She and her husband are much happier in their marriage, and oh yes, she is feeling so much better without the proverbial karmic monkey-wrench calling the shots for her.

A long-term follow up several years later revealed that she remained alcohol free for three full months and then resumed heavy drinking. I was fairly sure that she didn't utilize her protective God Light visualizations and affirmations as often as I had strongly suggested. I recommended that she come to see me or have me carry out a remote session on her with my assistant.

Beverly decided that she would like my assistant and me to carry out a remote entity releasement session, which we did, a few months later. This session revealed several dark force entities and two soul fragments which had previously been attached to alcoholics. The dark forces were removed and the soul fragments returned to their original souls. Soul fragments are very much like Earthbound spirits in that they are drawn to personalities with the same weakness, same issues, and same personality defects.

My assistant's Spirit Guide now began to speak. "Beverly has a very diminished self-worth and feels she's just not good enough. The dark forces contribute to these feelings in a very heavy fashion. Her husband, brother, and other relatives expect her to not do well, so she feels that she is just living up to their expectations. She is weary of trying to please others. She considers herself a failure when she drinks and experiences a void when she does not drink. She doesn't handle success well and finds that not feeling good about herself is easier to handle. Drinking fills the void and disconnects her from her feelings."

At this time I decided to ask my assistant's Spirit Guide if she had suggestions for Beverly that would help her. My assistant's Spirit Guide responded by saying, "Beverly needs to fill the void with something she enjoys, and also she needs to practice spiritual meditation. By doing so, she will attain peace and release the feeling of not being good enough. She must stop sabotaging herself by feeding the addiction of not feeling good enough with alcohol. Self-love and self-acceptance are the cure. We will send her Light and love."

Following the remote entity releasement session, I telephoned Beverly and filled her in on all the details of the session and once again encouraged her to carry out God Light visualization and affirmation in a consistent manner.

THE STUFF DREAMS ARE MADE OF

I would now like to focus on a specific segment of a case to point out one of the many ways Earthbound entities can interact with their host. This gentleman came to me with an array of physical problems as well as an obstruction to his progress in his professional life as an accountant. He said he felt that he had the gift of precognition both in the waking state and in the dream state. During the interview with this patient I discovered some very interesting symptoms that reeked of Earthbound spirit influence. One related to his doing just the opposite of what he intended to do. The other was the fact that before going to sleep he would be bombarded with other people's memories which always seemed to relate to the present time. On a few occasions he would be so irritated that he would shout, "Please leave me alone!"

His Spirit Guide was exceptionally helpful and assisted me in releasing much in the way of foreign energy. When we came to the presence of Earthbound spirits I was told that there were many and that they had all died in the patient's current lifetime. These Earthbound spirits had attached to the patient at different times for a temporary period of time for the purpose of completing unfinished business, and they did this by connecting through his dreams, making him a vessel. At that moment I remembered that he had foreknowledge of things to come in the dream state as well as in the waking state, and I thought to myself that this gift of precognition would be a tremendous help for Earthbound spirits who would now be able to immediately know the outcome of their unfinished business through the patient's foreknowledge of the future in his dream state. I then wondered if the patient's psychic gift of precognition was what attracted these Earthbound spirits in the first place. As it turned out, at least a dozen of these entities contributed to several of the patient's problems, and by removing them, I would be eliminating most of the patient's complaints. With this in mind I decided to assist all the Earthbound spirits in going to the Light and wished them Godspeed. In a follow up call several weeks later the patient told me that he feels good due to improvement in his physical problems and that he is no longer obstructed in making forward progress in his career.

LOVE KNOWS NO BOUNDARIES

Earthbound cases can involve gut-wrenching emotions for both the patient and the Earthbound spirit. I have run into many such cases and never cease to be amazed at the inner workings of the soul that contribute to the complexities of these cases.

One such case revolved around a young man who felt a deep connection to a woman who was twenty years younger that he is. Her name was Laura, and that name seemed to pop up everywhere, even in his dreams. He would hear voices saying, "Don't give up," and, "You hurt me." Under deep hypnosis the patient's Spirit Guide revealed the presence of an Earthbound spirit by the name of Garo. It seems that Garo was causing the patient to have fear, doubt, and an emptiness from the loss of a woman that Garo loved in a past lifetime. This was the only life that Garo had with this woman, and now she has returned in the patient's present life as Laura. I asked the patient's Spirit Guide to go back in time and give us an overview of the life that Garo had with Laura.

This lifetime occurred in ancient Greece where Garo was a member of the royal family. The woman in the patient's current life that the patient knows now as Laura was Garo's wife whom Garo loved very much in that life in ancient Greece. In that life she happened to be inspecting their many horses that were adorned with gold when thieves surprised her and stole the horses, taking Laura with them. Garo was fearful and did not go after the thieves, something he regretted all his life. His wife was never returned, and Garo died still looking for her.

Somehow Garo knew that the patient would eventually cross paths with Laura, and therefore he declined going to the Light, remained in the lower astral plane, and ultimately attached to the patient. I explained to Garo that his presence as an attached entity would not only be unsatisfying but rather uncomfortable for the patient and the woman known as Laura. I told him that it was important that he continue his spiritual journey by going to the Light and that he would be able to love her from the Light and eventually be able to share another lifetime with her in the future. He agreed, and I wished him Godspeed as he entered the Light.

I then turned my attention to the patient and asked his Spirit Guide if the patient also had a lifetime with this woman known as Laura. The answer I received was "Yes, several." I then requested that the Spirit Guide take us to those lifetimes for a brief overview of their togetherness.

The first lifetime showed the patient to be a 35-year-old male laborer whose only contact with Laura was a chance meeting in Germany. She was much older than he was, and he never got to know her in that lifetime. In a second lifetime with Laura he found himself in ancient Troy as a male in a white tunic. He had a brief relationship with her but no intimacy and eventually married some-one else. The patient was revealed to be a male farmer in a third life, and Laura was his younger sister, to whom he remained very close throughout their lives. The fourth lifetime took place in the pioneer days in the western United States. The patient was a male pioneer in a wagon train who became attracted to Laura, who was someone else's wife. The attraction was mutual and instantaneous, but the relationship was brief and ended in a very short time.

The patient's Spirit Guide felt the need to tell the patient that he, Garo, and Laura, are all from the same soul group and have made agreements in the afterlife. His advice to the patient was, "Be patient and pursue this relationship with Laura when the time is right; in other words, follow your heart."

THE EARTHBOUND SPIRIT THAT FELL IN LOVE

This young, single physician by the name of Elaine came to me with relationship issues and a rather unusual problem that had to do with her hearing voices at night while trying to go to sleep. The voices began approximately six months earlier, and the patient had tried to record them by placing a new recorder in her bedroom overnight. This was very unsuccessful, causing the patient to use an older recorder that she had, to see if for some reason it would pick up the voices. This older recorder had lots of static but was able to pick up the voices of a man and a child. It seemed as if the static was necessary for the voices to come through.

The several recordings that the patient made revealed many loving statements by a male voice which seemed to be solely directed to Elaine. The voices that were picked up also included that of a child who was often told by the male voice to be quiet. Elaine has also felt frequent light touches on her arms or legs during the day and sometimes during the night. Originally she was fearful but is no longer so and has told me that she feels somewhat fond of what seem to be spirits and has heard the male voice saying affectionate things to her which have led her to believe that he is being somewhat protective of her.

Once Elaine was taken into deep hypnosis I was able to locate and communicate with her Spirit Guide, who told me that the child was an attached Earthbound spirit of a six-year-old girl who drowned years earlier on the property which Elaine presently lives on. The male spirit, however, attached to Elaine well over six months ago and appears to control the little girl by telling her where to go and when to talk. This attached Earthbound male spirit also appears to have fallen in love with Elaine. The Spirit Guide became exceptionally quiet and then uttered, "I've detected several dark force entities attached to this male Earthbound spirit." I immediately performed an exorcism and removed the dark force entities. Following this I asked the patient's Spirit Guide to scan Elaine's frequencies for any further foreign energy. The Spirit Guide was unable to detect any and explained that Elaine had a visit in the past from an extraterrestrial, but there have been no attachments, implants, or abductions.

The Spirit Guide felt that the little girl's spirit should go to the Light. After helping this little spirit get to the Light and wishing her Godspeed, I then turned my attention to the male Earthbound spirit who said that he had died in 1970 at 38 years old after being shot. At that time he was single and was a laborer. He then spoke about the things he told Elaine, "I tell her sweet things... I'm not hurting her, and I would never leave her. I keep her company." He continued with statements that indicated a great affection for Elaine.

At that moment the patient's Spirit Guide recommended, "I think he should stay for now. Elaine needs the support and love at this time in her life and has already promised this Earthbound spirit that he could stay if he's not evil." The Spirit Guide continued, "He has been kind of bad, but Elaine is forgiving. He has had no lifetimes with her; still, he does not remember ever loving anyone like he loves Elaine." Instructions in protection and powerful suggestions were then given to the patient, who awakened from hypnosis with a big smile and a peaceful disposition.

VENGEFUL EARTHBOUND SPIRITS

Janet flew in from Sarasota, Florida, to see me several years after I had seen her for a multitude of problems. During her previous sessions I uncovered a large number of dark forces, Earthbound spirits, and soul fragments, most of whom were responsible for the many problems that she was experiencing. The remaining issues, according to the Spirit Guide, were related to present and past life events that were revealed to her at that time. The patient's soul was found to be severely fragmented, so a soul retrieval was also carried out at that time.

Janet felt that her previous sessions were the reason that she was improved and able to successfully stop using a powerful pain medication; however, in doing so, she encountered a severe form of insomnia which has caused her great suffering and has kept her from having a good night's sleep for a very long time.

Her hypnotic induction went smoothly, and her Spirit Guide checked her energy frequencies carefully and identified a lot of foreign energy, which included many dark forces and powerful dark forces, which were removed by a successful exorcism. Two Earthbound spirits were discovered, so I began to interview them. When the first Earthbound was asked to say his name, I just heard an abrupt, "No," and I immediately asked the Spirit Guide if dark forces were attached to this Earthbound spirit. The Spirit Guide's positive response was followed with a repeat exorcism, after which the Earthbound spirit's hostility dwindled somewhat. My interrogation revealed a vendetta that this Earthbound spirit had for the patient. His answer in response to my asking about his purpose in joining Janet was, "Fun and to enjoy making her life very difficult. My life with her over a thousand years ago was of no consequence. She was my slave; she was always afraid and would not submit, causing me to not be able to sleep. Now she is not to sleep. She should be serving me, not sleeping."

A second Earthbound spirit was also contributing to Janet's insomnia. He was her husband in a past life, who blamed her for the drowning death of their two-year-old child. Both Earthbound spirits had joined her sometime following her previous sessions, and both agreed to go to the Light with my help. The remaining foreign energy picked up by the Spirit Guide consisted of one attached extraterrestrial, who said his purpose in joining Janet was to observe her influence and see if that influence can be helpful to his species, a form of Grays. By answering my questions this extraterrestrial admitted that he was carrying out mind experiments by putting pressure on the part of her brain that controls inhibitions. This alien also admitted that she had one of his implants attached to her pineal gland and that she has been abducted on several occasions, at which time eggs were taken in order to create hybrids. He then told me that he has remained attached to Janet for many years and had successfully kept his frequency hidden during her previous sessions so he would not be discovered.

At that moment I asked the Spirit Guide if dark forces were also attached to this Gray extraterrestrial. I received an affirmative answer and immediately decided to not give this Gray an opportunity to hide or escape while I am removing dark force entities and then convincing him to remove his implant and leave; rather, I conducted an immediate exorcism and asked St. Michael the Archangel to take this extraterrestrial, his attached dark force entities, and his implant, to that special place in the Light where he takes them.

The patient was now free of foreign energy per her Spirit Guide; however, he now informed me that her soul was severely fragmented. The patient then underwent an extensive soul retrieval, making her now a complete soul.

During the remaining time in the hypnotic session the patient was again instructed in God Light visualization and affirmations so as to ward off further entity infestation and reminded to avoid conditions that increase vulnerability to such attachments. Powerful suggestions regarding pain and insomnia followed.

The following day the patient informed me that she had slept deeply and uninterrupted all night, something she hasn't done in a very long time. She also said this was the best night's sleep that she ever had.

STRONG PERSONALITIES COMING THROUGH

Myra was a twenty-eight-year-old woman from New Hampshire who had been struggling with excesses in eating, smoking, and drinking on weekends for many years.

She said she was able to reverse the situation several years ago and was proud of her accomplishment; however for the past month she has fallen back into the old destructive behavior and feels that this has also caused her to be judgmental and easily angered.

Her hypnotic induction went smoothly, and I was easily able to communicate with a valid and astute Spirit Guide who was eager to help me come up with answers for this very nice and very concerned patient. Her Spirit Guide, who had been with Myra for many lifetimes, checked the frequencies surrounding the patient and declared that the patient had foreign energy which consisted of only two Earthbound spirits.

I asked the first Earthbound spirit to please step forward and tell me his name and his purpose in joining Myra. The Earthbound spirit responded, "My name is Sam. I needed to hang out, so I joined

Myra." I then asked him how long he had been attached to Myra, and to please tell me about himself. Sam immediately came forth with, "I joined her at work a few months ago. I died in 1974 in a car accident when I was 17." I then prodded Sam with more questions regarding Myra's problems, to which he answered, "Yeah, I drink a lot of booze, and I liked to smoke… so what! I never ate that much, and oh yeah, I got pissed off easily and would get into fights which I usually won."

My suspicions regarding the cause of my patient's recent return to old habits and a sudden need for anger management were falling into place, but it wasn't until I heard this Earthbound spirit say that he joined her less than two months ago that I was convinced that he was the main cause of her recent problems. Her Spirit Guide agreed and said he was the main cause of Myra's addiction to alcohol and tobacco.

I found the second Earthbound to be gentle and cooperative. He said his name was Kyle, and he died at ten years old from an illness and joined the patient when she was four years old. She was close by in the hospital that he died in. Further questioning revealed that he was somewhat obese and was often teased in his childhood. It seems that he liked to eat. This attached entity easily accounts for the patient's ongoing problem with weight and probably for her starting to overeat again since her other bad habits had been reinstituted.

Myra was one of a minority of patients that allowed the full personality of the attached entities to come through her. The changes in her voice and the gruffness that came through Myra were unbelievable. It was as if the entities were in front of me and speaking directly to me. I now explained to both Earthbound spirits that they need to continue their spiritual journey by going to the Light and that I would be happy to help them do this. Both agreed, and I wished them both Godspeed as they entered the Light. Myra began to cry as Kyle left.

The Spirit Guide informed me that Kyle's influence upon Myra's appetite had haunted Myra for most of her life. He also said that several episodes of trauma that Myra had encountered in her lifetime had resulted in a fragmentation of her soul. I performed a soul retrieval, making her once more a complete soul, and followed with protective instructions to prevent future entity attachment. I then asked her Spirit Guide if any past lifetimes have contributed to her problems. I received a resounding, "No!" I completed the session by planting very powerful suggestions into Myra's subconscious mind in regard to smoking, drinking excessive alcohol, and extreme overeating. A follow up call some time later revealed that the patient felt good, lighter, and had more energy. In addition, she was no longer in the destructive behavior pattern of excesses in smoking, eating, or drinking alcohol. Several months later she still felt enthusiastic about the work that I do.

In addition to the clarity of personality that comes through when an Earthbound spirit is being interviewed, I would like to point out that this particular case also exemplifies the rapidity with which an Earthbound spirit can influence its host and also the fact that Earthbound spirits are like soul fragments in that they are drawn to a host with similar likes, addictions, and experiences.

FAMILY REUNION

Roger was a 32-year-old architect from Charlottesville, Virginia, who made an appointment with me to see if I could diagnose and hopefully cure him of worrisome physical problems. These problems began several years ago, following the death of his father. They consisted of infrequent chest pain and headaches and occasionally feeling a swirling sensation in his head. He has seen several medical specialists who have been unable to come up with a diagnosis, all of which has resulted in chronic anxiety, for which he is on medication.

Following hypnotic induction, I initially was unable to have a Spirit Guide come forward; however, I found myself communicating with the soul fragment of a teenaged boy. This soul fragment recently separated from his soul due to the trauma that occurred when he was accidentally shot by a friend. He said he felt rather confused and lost when he first joined Roger, but at the same time he was made to feel somewhat comfortable because of the rather pleasant group of souls who had already attached to Roger. I decided to ask this young soul fragment if he could help me identify those who have attached to Roger. He agreed and said Roger had six Earthbound spirits attached to him.

At this time I began to ask each Earthbound spirit to please step forward, tell me about themselves, and let me know if they had any of Roger's symptoms present when they were alive. As I interviewed each Earthbound spirit, it became obvious that Roger's family was drawn to him. Five of the six Earthbound spirits were from family members who had died. This included the souls of his parents, his godmother, two uncles, and a woman who joined him when he was a boy. Four of these entities admitted that they had some of Roger's symptoms present when they were alive, and these symptoms encompassed all of Roger's complaints.

At this point I once again called for a Spirit Guide, who now responded. His name was Jim, he accepted Light, and I felt that he was extremely valid. All the Earthbound spirits were agreeable to going to the Light to continue their spiritual journey. I helped them get to the Light and wished them Godspeed. I then did a soul retrieval and returned our teenaged soul fragment to his original soul. Following confirmation of all this by the Spirit Guide, he picked up on the frequency of one dark force who had been trying to attach to Roger for some time but has not been successful. An exorcism was performed and confirmed, after which the Spirit Guide announced that Roger had no further foreign energy, was not fragmented, and no past lifetimes had contributed to his issues. The Spirit Guide wanted me to know that Roger will definitely see improvement in his physical problems and also felt that I should know that Roger had only lived three lifetimes and is slated to eventually become a Master Spirit. When I heard this, I thought the purpose of lifetimes is to learn lessons, so very possibly Roger may have learned most of his lessons.

Chapter 7

EXTRATERRESTRIALS

Astronomers estimate that the universe contains billions of galaxies, most of which are composed of more than a billion stars, some of which are solar systems. Earth is an integral part of our solar system that lies within the Milky Way galaxy, which contains some 300 billion stars. Earth-sized planets in other solar systems within our galaxy have been found to be located in a habitable zone. Skeptics will often scoff at the possibility of extraterrestrial presence. The history of mankind is replete with all kinds of evidence of extraterrestrial visitation. To think that we are alone in this endless universe speaks of the stubborn narrow-mindedness of such skeptics.

According to Master Spirits, most souls will choose to incarnate on Earth rather than on other planets because if a lesson is truly learned on Earth, it is learned very well. However, life on Earth is not easy, and after many attempts to learn lessons in different lifetimes on Earth, some of which are successful, and some of which are not successful, the soul may feel the need for a less stressful life, which I understand from various patients exists on many planets. According to these patients, the planets they refer to are without disease or war and have an extended longevity.

(Once again, I feel the need to step back and objectively look over everything that I am saying to the reader. Over twenty-three years ago, as a conventional physician I would have been shocked at what I am presenting here; however, at the same time, that conventional part of me is impressed with the fact that all the information that I have received has come from the subconscious minds of thousands of patients, and the consistency of content is overwhelming. More importantly, the therapeutic value is massive, and as a physician, I feel compelled to pass on what my research has taught me. The material that follows is no exception.)

My research is astonishing in that I am able to communicate with these non-human entities through my patients. I suspect that extraterrestrials have the technology to be able to go from a physical dimension into a spirit-like dimension, and thus cannot be seen by humans. This non-physical form apparently allows them to attach to and influence humans without their knowledge. I find that extra-terrestrials are very candid and are usually willing to communicate and explain what they are doing. Occasionally I run into hostile extraterrestrials who are not so willing to explain their presence. When this occurs I will immediately ask the patient's Spirit Guide to check for dark force attachments on the extraterrestrials. If dark forces are attached to these alien beings, I will perform an exorcism and remove them. Once this is completed, the extraterrestrial is usu-ally quite amenable to understanding the situation and is coopera-tive as far as detaching from the patient and returning to his home planet. I have come upon extraterrestrial species who are benevolent, some who are inherently hostile, namely, some of the Grays, and others who are basically demonic, primarily the Reptilians. All of these various species of extraterrestrials have communicated with me through many patients.

A common thread regarding visits by extraterrestrials is that they will often make their visits at a person's home late at night; however, they may come at any time and thus be responsible for missing time in locations where the person is alone, or with others who will also experience this strange rearrangement of time.

Most abducted patients complain of missing time, low energy, nighttime paralysis, and occasionally, fear of flying. I have come across several patients who, while under deep hypnosis, said that they felt themselves floating through walls and being sucked up into a flying ship. Many of these patients recognized and understood why they have this fear of flying, as they almost instantly related this fear of flying to flying in a ship with these non-human beings. Once they arrived in this ship, they found themselves imprisoned in a sterile room whereupon strange looking beings appeared to be performing abdominal surgical procedures on them. (The descriptions I have been given of what took place in those sterile rooms very much resemble laparoscopic procedures on a patient's abdomen utilizing a scope designed to go through a tiny skin opening, usually adjacent to and below the umbilicus. In modern medicine, these scopes utilize a fiber optic technique to light the area for the surgeon.) Some of these patients recall hearing comments about removing eggs or placement of implants, and at the same time, sense a strong energy frequency bombarding their body while telepathically hearing, "You won't remember."

During hypnotic sessions, the Reptilians have told me that they hate the Light, despise Light Workers, and as often as possible interrupt the Light Workers' mission of bringing Light and love to the inhabitants of various planets. I have had many patients who are considered Light Workers on Earth. Some of them were also Light Workers on other planets before incarnating on Earth. The Reptilians do not mind telling me that their agenda is to conquer as many planets as they can. They accomplish this by implanting devices and other means. Reptilians are unable to manipulate Light Workers due to the amount of Light within them; however, they will attempt to control them as much as possible by placing implants within them. Light Workers are able to remove these implants, so

Reptilians often send robots to ensure that the implants remain in place.

Reptilians have also informed me through various patients that Light Workers from Sirius and other planets built the pyramids on Earth and placed crystals within them. When asked about reproduction among Reptilians, I was told that they are not interested in sex because they don't want more Reptilians to share with. They followed with, "We don't want love, just power." I've also had some cases where a Reptilian hybrid will meet a Light Worker and develop an emotional bond with him so as to distract him from his purpose. I've also been told by the three-fingered Reptilian species that they have abducted Light Workers on Earth and other planets and are able to conduct emotional and spiritual experiments upon them.

AN EXTRATERRESTRIAL DESCRIBES HIS METHOD OF ATTACHMENT

During an interview with one of my patients whom I will call Paul, I was informed that at the age of thirteen he had a very lucid dream wherein he saw himself being shot in the back with a gun. The following night he had a similar dream, but this time he was shot with an arrow in that same location. When taken back to the cause of this recurring dream, Paul began seeing beings that were not like people. He described them as being roughly eight feet tall, with thin bodies, long arms, and large heads. At that moment the patient's Spirit Guide interrupted and explained that these beings were a group of twelve aliens who appeared to be doing something to Paul's back. I then asked to communicate to whoever was in charge of the extraterrestrials and asked what they were doing. He answered, "I am attaching myself by placing a one-inch wide by six-inch long organic tubular structure into a specific area in this person's back. It is just to the left of his vertebrae and seven vertebrae up from the bottom vertebral bone. This tube grabs on to skin and muscle, and the attachment is then carried out through an energy transfer within our dimension. At the time, Paul is stunned or frozen by this energy, so he does not feel pain. Only one of us is attached; the others here just feel his energy." The Spirit Guide once again interrupted and said that the insertion of the alien's organic tube was in the identical spot in his back in which Paul had been shot in his dreams.

I have heard of various other forms of attachment performed by extraterrestrials, and I have a feeling that they are species-specific; I have found that whenever there is a group of extraterrestrials present, there usually is only one that is attached, and that is usually the leader.

The alien in charge again spoke and said, "We are Grays from the planet Niberu, sent to watch over Paul. Paul had been one of us until he decided to incarnate on Earth, his first incarnation as a human. We are here to make him feel better and not have feelings of loneliness. Paul hates it here."

When I asked the alien leader for a description of life on Niberu, I was told that it is bigger than Earth, mostly green, and has a population of around 80,000. Reproduction is through thought energy; longevity is around eighty years old; and there are no wars. Communication is telepathic, their diet consists of mostly greens, and their digestive track is similar to humans; however, the mouth and anus are smaller. The Spirit Guide corroborated that the patient had never been on Earth before, had three lifetimes on Niberu, and had 87 lives on other planets. The guide also said that the Grays' 80-year longevity is actually 800 Earth years; and following death, their souls ascend to the Light, which is a bluish color. (I have found that the color of the afterlife varies considerably with different planets.) Paul's Spirit Guide felt that these extraterrestrials should not have to leave since they are not causing any problem and are in fact helping Paul feel better about his life on Earth.

Sometime after this most interesting session I received an email from this patient. He wanted me to know that his life has improved immensely since our session, and he feels like he knows who he is and understands life on Earth so much better. He also said that he would like to return for another session and learn more about his many lifetimes on other planets.

THE BENEVOLENT REPTILIAN

A patient by the name of Henry told me that a psychic reading revealed that he had been a pilot for a spaceship from the planet Sirius. This patient subsequently had a past life regression with another hypno-therapist wherein Henry saw himself as a benevolent humanoid-type Reptilian, with a human type face, velvety skin, and an abundance of emotions, including love and a strong sense of justice. He was cap-tured by evil Reptilians from the same planet and taken to another planet, where he was sold and kept in captivity, a dimension of dark-ness. Later this patient had a spontaneous conscious flashback and he felt himself in that Reptilian body. He also recognized someone in his present life to be the evil Reptilian leader who had made him suffer in that lifetime. The suffering was so intense that part of his soul fragmented and still remains in that dark prison.

When Henry came to see me, I attempted and completed a soul retrieval by requesting that several Archangels march into that dark place and rescue his soul fragment which was then returned and integrated into the patient's existing soul, giving him a feeling of being complete. Henry felt that the evil Reptilian leader was very much influenced by dark forces. I encouraged forgiveness of this presently-embodied reincarnation of the evil Reptilian. Once that was accomplished, the patient felt a great weight being lifted from him.

RELEASING A LIGHT WORKER'S GIFTS

This patient was a 32-year-old woman from Great Britain who felt that she has had experiences with extraterrestrials for many years.

She described a time when extraterrestrials who appeared to be Grays caused her to be paralyzed while they took her son away for a short time. Following hypnotic induction, I was able to communicate with her Spirit Guide and carried out an exorcism of several dark force entities, including a powerful one. When it came to identifying the frequencies of extraterrestrials, the guide was unsure, so I called for a more experienced Spirit Guide, who came forth and immediately identified a total of seven extraterrestrials from two separate species. At that moment the patient felt a heavy pressure on her chest and woke up. I quickly carried out a rapid re-induction, took the patient deep, and once again attempted to communicate with the Spirit Guides. To my amazement and disappointment the patient remained silent. At this juncture I had no doubt that dark forces were somehow involved, in spite of the fact that I had just removed them. I felt that they woke the patient up and created an obstruction to the further release of entities from outer space. I was confused, but I knew I was dealing with something dark and needed to resort to extreme measures, one of which I have used successfully before. Using it again, I spoke the words, "I hereby invoke the help of St. Michael the Archangel to please blast a path through the obstruction so Spirit Guides may get through." Within seconds the Spirit Guide responded through the patient and confirmed that one of the extraterrestrial species was Reptilian, a very demonic Reptilian. I quickly performed an exorcism and had St. Michael the Archangel take all the Reptilians, attached and unattached, to the special place in the Light that he takes them.

Following confirmation of this successful exorcism, the patient's Spirit Guide began describing the other species as one that was benevolent. I asked to speak to their leader, and to my surprise I began to hear giggles as a voice then said, "We are all leaders."

I asked the name of their species and their purpose in being here.

He replied, "I am unable to translate the name of our species into your language; however you can call us 'Keepers.' We are Light Beings and we are here to interfere with the demonic Reptilians.

They have taken over many planets but at the cost of many lives we were able to keep them from taking over our planet."

I then asked, "Why have the Reptilians decided to cause problems for my patient?"

He answered, "The Reptilians knew she was a Light Worker and bound her gifts so she was unable to use her Light. They did not do experiments on her and were unsuccessful at trying to manipulate her. Her Light prevented such control." (I have heard this many times before from other patients.) "They, however, did place an implant within her so that whenever she used her Light, it would bring Reptilians to her."

Hearing this I immediately asked for St. Michael the Archangel to take the implant to the Light. Following confirmation of the implant removal, the patient's Spirit Guide said that these benevolent extraterrestrials were not attached, and it was okay for them to stay and keep an eye on the patient and prevent further Reptilian interference.

Following further work under hypnosis, including instruction in God Light visualization and affirmation, the patient was awakened and immediately said that during the invocation of St. Michael the Archangel to blast a path through the obstruction, she felt a small area within the center of her chest begin to open and release some of the pressure. This was followed by an explosive feeling in her chest as the pressure seemed to be suddenly forced out of her chest, giving her great relief, a feeling of freedom, and allowing her Spirit Guide to once again communicate.

LIGHT IS STRENGTH

I have heard many Spirit Guides describe a patient's abduction by extraterrestrials. One young woman's Spirit Guide spoke of multiple abductions by Reptilians wherein the patient was taken while sleeping and brought to the mother ship where she was raped, and eggs were removed from her. The Spirit Guide said the Reptilians not only took her spirit of joy away but also tried to control her and have her do their bidding. Fortunately, she was a Light Worker with an exceptional amount of Light within her, making her entirely too strong for them to control her. The Spirit Guide concluded with the fact that this patient had many lifetimes on other planets and just one life as a benevolent Reptilian on their planet.

NOT ALL EXTRATERRESTRIALS ARE GOOD SURGEONS

As long as we are on the subject of extraterrestrial abdominal scoping and removal of eggs, I would like to mention a case involving a patient in her early eighties who told me that one morning some forty years ago she woke up with umbilical pain. When she looked at her umbilicus, she was stunned to see a scar that had changed the shape of her umbilicus. This area was somewhat reddish and swollen and remained uncomfortable for several weeks. The patient said her gynecologist had performed a diagnostic laparoscopy on her abdomen through her umbilicus ten years before that and left a very fine scar that was barely perceptible. (I have done many of these procedures and have closed the laparoscopic incision with subcuticular stitches, leaving virtually no scar.) Thus this rather hideous-looking scar that the patient was observing that morning was new. The patient showed me her umbilical scar, and I could definitely see both vertical and horizontal scars that were quite obvious. I thought to myself that laparoscopy scars are barely, if ever, perceptible, and that the extraterrestrials who performed this scoping were either poorly trained or ran into problems and had to widen the incision to get more exposure. I have no other way to explain this painful and rather extensive scarring that the patient discovered that morning.

THE PATIENT FROM CENTAURI

Christine was a thirty-year-old patient who had developed an incessant form of insomnia some seven months prior to the appointment. The insomnia seemed to take place in the middle of the night. Christine went on to describe several bizarre occurrences that she had been experiencing. These included missing time, an ability to feel energy and see unusual auras, and having knowledge of certain things before they happen. In addition, she was having problems with her marriage.

Following hypnotic induction, Christine went very deep into hypnosis and was able to summon her Spirit Guide, who turned out to be extremely helpful. When asked to take the patient back to the cause of her insomnia the Spirit Guide had Christine see thousands of stars and galaxies and finally a planet named Centauri which was three light years away.

The Guide then said, "Right now you are visiting Earth; Centauri is your real home. The time is coming when there will be a massive nuclear explosion with much devastation. A ship from Centauri will be coming to take you back where you belong before this happens. You are being called at night and communicated with telepathically. Your gifts are from Centauri. You are not enjoying sex and therefore don't need it. It does not compare with the energy you received from your partner during sexual intimacy on Centauri, which resulted in a child. Since you chose to have a life on Earth, Centaurians planted a child in you while you were asleep at the age of seventeen."

I interrupted and asked Christine's Spirit Guide to show her how conception took place. Almost instantly Christine's Spirit Guide began to describe seeing a four and a half foot alien male reach for Christine's hand while she slept. At that moment she could actually feel an unbelievably pleasurable feeling of energy which she remembered when she woke up that morning, and the feeling lasted for days. She also remembered that for several days she could smell something unusual but at the same time it was familiar.

Christine's Spirit Guide explained that the energy and sperm transferred together. He then said, "Several weeks later you began to bleed on and off and became very sick for four days. Those who came from Centauri took the fetus while you slept and grew it in a laboratory. Your son is pure Centaurian. He comes to you in dreams and is waiting for you to come home."

I saw the patient in a follow up appointment over a year later. At that visit she informed me that her insomnia problem disappeared within days of her first appointment.

EXTRATERRESTRIALS THAT ARE NEITHER EVIL NOR BENEVOLENT

Occasionally I run into an extraterrestrial that is obstinate, argumentative, and not compassionate. I find that this particular type of extraterrestrial is not demonic and does not have a dark force attached to it. The patient's physical description of the extraterrestrial resembles that of the Grays. These extraterrestrials have their orders and intend to carry them out, thus completing their mission. If I request that this form of alien being remove any implants and return to his planet, he will either refuse to leave or try intimidation. I normally do not treat this type of extraterrestrial as I would a dark force entity or evil Reptilian, which would entail a full exorcism and removal by St. Michael the Archangel.

A case in point involves a young woman who came to me complaining of depression and excesses in drinking and smoking. When this patient was attempting to go to sleep at eight years old, she momentarily saw an egg shaped face leaning over her, which caused her to scream. Later she had a traumatic dream in her late teens that was followed by nighttime paralysis. During this paralysis she was hearing voices which were giving technical information which was difficult to comprehend, and at the same time she was having feelings of being not where she was supposed to be. All this had made it hard for her to move forward in life. Under deep hypnosis, she began to recall dreams where she felt herself being aboard a flying ship in a room with blue lights, where curious beings were seeking information about her feelings, emotions, and sexuality. In another dream she found herself inside a sterile room with a long instrument protruding from her left lower abdomen. She felt that these beings were somehow removing eggs from her.

Using Abel, the volunteer Spirit Guide who spoke through the patient, I uncovered an array of Earthbound spirits, many of whom were smokers and drinkers, several dark force entities, and a very elusive and cocky extraterrestrial, with whom I had a long confrontation.

The attachments really had the patient buffaloed, as she kept saying things like, "I'm not good enough", and, "I'll feel empty if they leave." Finally I accomplished what was needed by removing all the dark force entities and Earthbound spirits and by convincing the cocky extraterrestrial to leave. If my efforts to rid the patient of this obnoxious extraterrestrial had been unsuccessful, I would have conducted an exorcism to carry this out. The session came to an end after carrying out protective instructions and powerful suggestions.

THE ALIEN COLONIST

A few years ago I encountered an extraterrestrial who was stubborn but not hostile. Dr. William Baldwin has named these types of extraterrestrials "alien colonists" and felt that they are intent on expanding their reach and establishing colonized outposts on other planets. He says they attach so as to exert some degree of control over people's minds. I agree with Dr. Baldwin, that they are quite arrogant in regard to their superiority and generally refuse to leave.

A woman in her mid-60s came to see me with chronic upper back pain. The patient also had been on medication for schizophrenic episodes and bipolar behavior for many years. I discovered an extraterrestrial attachment, and when I asked about his purpose in being here, the extraterrestrial responded, "I feed off her energy."

I asked, "Where?"

He replied, "Her upper back." He then volunteered the fact that he also did mind experiments on this person. I immediately thought to myself that this may be the reason for her schizophrenia and bipolarity.

My initial attempts at convincing this alien to leave were unsuccessful because the ET did not understand or care about his uninvited intrusion causing this person to suffer. I then used one of Dr. Baldwin's techniques, which was to ask the ET if his planet had ever been invaded, and if so, how did that make him feel. The next step was to relate this scenario to the problems that the ET's invasive experiments were causing in the patient. The extraterrestrial finally understood and agreed to leave.

Follow up several months later found the patient to be pain-free and no longer requiring medications, since she no longer had any symptoms of back pain, schizophrenia, or bipolarity.

THE DECEPTIVE ANDROID

Francine was a 37-year-old actress who was suffering from anxiety, depression, drug-addiction, relationship problems, and a constant feeling that she deserved to be punished. Her Spirit Guide came forth following her hypnotic induction and was exceptionally helpful. The Guide immediately let Francine know that she had over 100 lifetimes, some of which were with her current boyfriend. In regard to her relationship problems with her boyfriend, the Spirit Guide advised that she was not to pursue it for now. He felt that her boyfriend needs to grow up and she needs to let go for now and understand that the future may be different.

Francine's Spirit Guide revealed the presence of many dark force entities and one extraterrestrial. The dark force entities were removed without incident, leaving the one extraterrestrial, who said that he has been with Francine since she was a child and that he was compassionate and watches over her. The extraterrestrial said that he was an android (i.e., a machine or robot) from Uranus, who did things that made Francine happy and showed her what's possible. With his help she could turn lights on with her thoughts, read peoples' energy and control energy with her mind, enabling her to heal people. Francine used this psychic gift to heal a paralyzed relative who was then able to walk.

As I listened to this glowing report of compassion and helpfulness, I thought to myself, "So why does she have all these problems?" I decided to interrupt the extraterrestrial by asking Francine's Spirit Guide if this extraterrestrial had done any experimentation on Francine.

Her Spirit Guide suddenly voiced his irritation as he blurted out, "The extraterrestrial won't show himself to me!" I then asked the Spirit Guide again to tell us if experiments were carried out, and if they were, to describe them.

Francine's Spirit Guide answered by saying, "Yes, the extraterrestrial did experiments whereupon he would etherically use his fingers on her chest and thus look into her chest and mind. This resulted in her self-punishment." There was a moment of silence, and then the Spirit Guide cried out, "The extraterrestrial is gone!" At that moment Francine became somewhat emotional and said she felt very different.

Her Spirit Guide continued, "The extraterrestrial had been keeping me from being by Francine's side by sending her a heavy energy which has kept her from enjoying her childhood. Francine just wanted to have a good time in a good way. She just wanted to be happy. The extraterrestrials' experiments made her feel that she deserved to be punished and kept her depressed a good part of the time. Her parents were the cause of her anxiety and also contributed to her depression. The dark forces made everything worse by causing her to have dark thoughts and a dark contemplation of death. Francine needs to make up her mind and choose to stop taking drugs and stay off of them."

I followed by stressing the importance of God Light visualization and affirmation and gave powerful suggestions to the subconscious in regard to anxiety, depression, self-esteem, drug addiction, and relationships. In a follow up phone call several days later Francine told me that she was doing well on all fronts.

THE PINK PLANET

You, the reader, have had a taste of what extraterrestrial lives are all about, as they enter the domain of human experience for purposes of curiosity, observation, experimentation, control, or just to keep an eye on those who came from their planet. Let's now take a brief look at what life is like on another planet.

In my first book, *From Birth to Rebirth*, I wrote about a patient's description of what life is like in another galaxy. The patient was a young woman who had several traumatic past lifetimes, so I thought it would be a good idea to have her regress to her happiest and most peaceful lifetime. She soon found herself living a past life on another planet in a faraway star system. The planet was described as being pink all the time due to a gaseous vapor which was generated from the ocean water. There was no day or night, and the temperature remained comfortable and never varied. An intricate description of the inhabitants, who were mostly pink in color, was related to me in great detail. This planet allowed the inhabitants to live long, happy, peaceful lives, since the planet was without war and without disease; however, according to the patient, life was rather boring since the planet was also without music or other forms of entertainment. I have heard similar descriptions of other planets which reinforces my thoughts regarding the fact that Earth is a tough place, with its long history of war and disease, but it definitely is more exciting and certainly not boring.

Sometime after my first book was published, I received an email from an enlightened reader who told me he had just finished reading *From Birth to Rebirth*. He wanted me to know my description of a planet in the chapter entitled "Life on Other Planets" validated several visions that were related to memories that he could not explain nor understand. He told me he had visions of what he called *The Pink Planet*, the portrayal of which was almost identical to what I described in my book. This included details regarding the appearance of the inhabitants as well. He ended the email by saying that he now feels good, knowing this vision was not just his imagination.

THE ORIGINAL ATLANTIS

In my book *From Birth to Rebirth*, I talk about the consistency of past life memories observed by different patients in regard to the destruction of the lost continent of Atlantis. I continue to see patients who, according to their Spirit Guides, have had lives in Atlantis, and I find that there is also a consistency in the reporting that extraterrestrials were involved in the formation of Atlantis. The following case adds more dimension to that last statement.

When a young male patient told me he had always been intrigued by Mystery Schools and felt that he had lived in Atlantis, I was compelled to take him back to that life. Following induction and the acquisition of a helpful Spirit Guide, the patient found himself on the planet Tara, working in a laboratory, observing a fish in a tank. He was a 30-year-old male who was the director of a scientific project involving DNA strings. His colleagues in this laboratory were extraterrestrials from other star systems. He described them as tall with smooth skin and cone shaped heads. These individuals were experienced in that they had built many pyramids here, which served as energy sources. This area of Tara is called Atlantis and has many portals, energy sources, and stations for ships to be launched into space. The remaining area of Tara is controlled by the Nemurians, who have the majority of the crystals on the planet that were acquired by forceful acquisition. The Atlanteans wanted their crystals back, and a war ensued, causing massive explosions which eventually destroyed the planet. Some Atlanteans escaped by spaceship and founded an area on Earth which they called Atlantis. The patient's Spirit Guide interjected that the patient had three lifetimes on the original Atlantis, fifty lifetimes on other planets, and

72 lifetimes so far on Earth, including one in Sumer. The Spirit Guide also informed me that the patient had attachments that were soul fragments from the Atlantis on Tara. One was humanoid, the other non-humanoid.

CONSTRUCTION OF THE PYRAMIDS

I find that I never tire from the surprises that I encounter around every corner. These surprises are in reality gifts of valuable information that come from the subconscious minds of patients. A young woman from Chicago made an appointment to see if I could help her overcome Tourette syndrome. With the help of a very capable Spirit Guide, I was able to take her back to the cause of her Tourette syndrome. Her subconscious mind turned out to be a treasure trove of information regarding extraterrestrial activity that occurred in antiquity.

She went back to a life in ancient Egypt. She was a male by the name of Beta in that lifetime and arrived in northern Egypt on a shuttle from a large spaceship at the age of three. The spaceship was occupied by nearly 100 other humanoids, individuals that were genetically modified so that they would look very much like humans. Their spaceship came from a faraway star system and carried a large amount of equipment. The patient sensed that Beta was born on the mother ship, which was growing hybrids and taking them to Earth for the purpose of constructing pyramids. The hybrids were sent at a very young age so they would be able to adjust and acclimate to the planet Earth. A few adults were sent with them to help them adjust and eventually instruct them in regard to the specific jobs that they had and get them started.

When Beta was 23 years old in that lifetime, he found himself piloting a specially-designed flying vehicle that had come with his shuttle. This flying machine was one of several that hovered and was capable of attaching, lifting, and carrying the massive rock slabs that were used to construct the pyramids. He piloted this single-manned hovering vehicle for many years. When I asked how this technologically-advanced machine accomplished this feat, the patient's Spirit Guide said it used a form of anti-gravity energy which penetrated the entire thickness of the rock and connected to the spaceship shuttle, making the rock an extension of the ship. The massive rock slabs were meticulously placed into predetermined positions with great precision. Egyptians were used to clean up and work on the inside of the pyramids, which had a source of light. Beta was also aware of many roomy openings inside the pyramid and a large crystal that reflected light. The patient's Spirit Guide said that in that life very few of Beta's fellow humanoid workers knew the purpose of the pyramids. When he was 23, two thirds of the construction had been completed, and the estimated Earth time for the construction was forty years.

At this point in the regression I asked the Spirit Guide if Beta had made any inquiries regarding the purpose of the pyramids. The response was that Beta was not supposed to know and went on to describe what the individual who was overseeing the construction looked like. His description was that of a species that appeared as a cross between a human and a praying mantis.

When I questioned the patient's Spirit Guide with regard to the specific cause of the patient's Tourette syndrome, I was told that this syndrome was a characteristic that often occurs when one comes to Earth from another galaxy. The Tourette syndrome remained dormant during her life as a male in Egypt, as it did with the other humanoids, but a certain food triggered its appearance in her present life. At this moment the patient saw an orange in her mind's eye and intuitively knew she should stay away from oranges and their juice.

When I took another patient back to the cause of a recurring dream wherein he saw himself inside the Great Pyramid during its construction, I was astonished to hear a similar description of the construction process regarding the Great Pyramid in Giza. Under hypnotic regression and with the Spirit Guide's help, he again saw himself inside the Great Pyramid during its construction, during a life in ancient Egypt around 2500 BC. He was a spiritual ruler at that time. When the patient continued, I became very excited to hear statements which validated what I had heard before, namely that the very large stones were brought to the site and put into position with a flying vehicle that used a form of energy to lift and place the rocks. My excitement heightened when I heard that this was all accomplished with the help of friends of the Egyptians, who were described as "other life forms." I also was told that the Egyptian laborers worked primarily on the inside of the pyramid.

INTER-DIMENSIONAL BEINGS

I leave it to the Spirit Guides to identify the various entities that are attached, especially when it comes to extraterrestrials. Occasionally the Spirit Guide will point out that a very unusual type of being, who may be attached or unattached, is really an inter-dimensional being. I have since discovered that these beings vary considerably. Two such cases are described below.

HALF AND HALF

Once such being had the name "Avamar" and was described by the patient's Spirit Guide as "an extraterrestrial who visits." The name of his people was "Mantrex." He had been created to be partially mechanical and partially bioengineered living tissue and to have the ability to travel through time and space. He had been programmed to study this particular patient's biology and had discovered that this patient's DNA could be useful to his people, who did not carry out abductions or experimentation; instead, they believed in observation and study. According to the Spirit Guide, the presence of the inter-dimensional beings has been causing the patient to have abdominal discomfort. Avamar did not want to leave, so I asked St. Michael the Archangel to remove him.

NEVER TO BE BORN OR DIE

Another form of inter-dimensional being identified himself to a patient's Spirit Guide as "Zu" from "Rexon," which is a dimension, not a planet, and is located between parts of space. Zu said that he was an inter-dimensional being, an observer who was to collect data and experiences and share them with the community of beings in his dimension, which he described as a collective intelligence. He said this way he could enrich his community, the members of which often joined together to flow or blend with each other. He continued by telling the Spirit Guide, "We are always the same number. There is no birth or death; no males or females. We are red and orange with no fixed shape or mass, and we are always moving, changing, joining, separating, and going off to collect more experiences, especially those of a richer sense that deal with the depth of emotions and interactions. We also observe animals on Earth and on other planets. These observations are random and not planned. Gas seeps from one space to another. We have no choice of where we go. We are not a full consciousness. We are different due to the blending. We are more of a shared consciousness, a deep bottom of a well. We interact only with each other, not with humans."

Chapter 8

SOUL FRAGMENTS

A living person's soul, also referred to as mind or consciousness, may undergo a fragmentation as a result of emotional or physical trauma. These living fragments may not return to the person's soul and therefore remain in the lower astral plane, thus leaving this soul incomplete and extremely vulnerable to entity attachment, especially if there are many fragments missing.

If the separated fragment remains separated, it may attach to another living person and do what uninvited attached entities usually do, namely influence the patient/host with its thoughts and its problems. The soul fragment remains at the age it was when it separated from its primary soul; therefore, it has no memory of anything that occurs to the primary soul after that age. My experience has shown that the particular trauma or issues that the patient/host has been dealing with will act like a magnet and draw these soul fragments from living people because these soul fragments can identify with the same issues that the patient is experiencing. This situation is quite similar to Earthbound spirits being attracted for the same reasons.

When I discover these foreign-energy soul fragments attached to my patients, I will interview them much like I do the Earthbound spirits, and in doing so determine the effects that they are having on the patient and confirm this with the patient's Spirit Guide.

Following these interrogations I will ask the patient's Spirit Guide to help with a soul retrieval so these foreign soul fragments can be returned to their original, or primary, souls. I refer to this as "foreign-energy soul fragment retrieval," which includes a deportation of the foreign-energy soul fragment and a retrieval by its original soul. In the process I instruct the soul fragments to look for a silver thread leading away from them and follow it to their original soul, where it will reunite and be welcomed back. As the original soul embraces the fragment, gifts are exchanged. Gifts such as love and security will be given to the soul fragment by the original soul, who will receive in return gifts from the fragment, such as humor and lightheartedness. Thus each attached soul fragment is returned to the soul it originated from.

By the same token, the Spirit Guide is asked if the patient's soul has been fragmented, and how many times. If fragmentation has occurred, the patient is instructed to search for silver threads leading from hollow areas within his body. The patient is then told to follow the largest silver thread, and in the process, observe the traumatic event and re-experience the fragmentation and the emotions that occurred at that time. Dr. Baldwin's extensive experience with these types of patients concluded that if the trauma occurred when the patient was a young child, the young sub-personality needs to understand that it came through the traumatic incident okay, it did not die, and the patient is who it became. I feel that it is often necessary for the patient to forgive all those involved in the trauma, including himself, if needed, to fully resolve this traumatic memory. The patient is now further instructed to locate and pull back this and all the silver threads leading away from his body, thus allowing a soul retrieval to take place with a similar exchange of gifts, thus allowing a person to retrieve his own soul fragments. I refer to this as "host soul fragment retrieval." The patient emerges from this course of action feeling immensely better, knowing without reservation and with Spirit Guide confirmation that he is once again a complete soul and no longer as vulnerable as he was to parasitic entity infestation.

Sometimes soul fragments are from people in your current life who had past lives with you, leaving unfinished business from one or more of those past lives which relate to karmic debts. I have encountered patients who were obsessed with sex due to a rather libidinous soul fragment attached to them. Some of these cases involved soul fragments from a sexual predator. Once these soul fragments were removed and returned to their original souls through soul retrieval, the patient almost always displayed marked improvement in his or her sexual appetite. If that wasn't bad enough, I have also come across a patient with soul fragments from an individual who held great hatred for the patient and brought him an excessive amount of negative energy in the form of a curse. (The subject of curses is discussed in Chapter Four.) Supposedly, the massive amount of hatred that this individual had for the patient was traumatic enough to cause the soul of the person with this extreme hatred to fragment. Once the fragmentation took place, the fragment found the patient and attached to him. People who engage in this demonic behavior are usually involved in witchcraft or satanic cults and believe that fragmentation of their soul under these circumstances adds power to the curse.

All these problems with patients are magnified by the influence of attached dark forces, which contribute to the patient's depression, lack of self-esteem, and sexual dysfunction. I have further come upon a case of molestation by a priest and have surprisingly found soul fragments of the priest attached to the victim. It seems that these wayward priests are also undergoing a sort of trauma, knowing that they are committing very sinful and hurtful acts.

The Spirit Guide will always help identify the cause of the patients' problems and all too often the problems relate to attached soul fragments of people in the patients' present lives. Once these fragments of living people's souls are returned to their original souls by soul retrieval and other attached entities and curses are properly removed, the patient is pronounced free of foreign energy by his

Spirit Guide and is now instructed in God Light visualization and affirmation. When attached soul fragments are from a past lifetime, the patient is taken to that lifetime so as to uncover all aspects of the unfinished business in that life before the soul retrieval is performed.

Follow up weeks later in sexual dysfunction cases will often find the patient feeling lighter, having more energy, and having less sexual dysfunction and fewer negative thoughts. Once again I need to remind the reader that when the same actions are carried out for long periods of time, grooves are set in the brain tissue. Once the cause of the action is removed, the grooves will eventually flatten out, so recovery is slow but steady. Initial improvement is a good sign.

FEAR

Fear is often considered the most negative emotion that a human being can have, and we already know that it is one of the greatest, if not the greatest, weapon that is used by the dark forces. I remember an exemplary case involving Sheila, a young woman from the state of Oregon who presented with an array of fears which caused her to be barely able to move forward in life.

Sheila had lost her husband, Albert, several years earlier and has never recovered from his death. Also, her history includes a very poor childhood in which she received negative programming from her parents for many years. Her fearful stance has even affected her curiosity concerning her future, and so she is afraid of that as well. She also would panic at the thought of driving.

Sheila easily entered into deep hypnosis during her first session and had much in the way of foreign energy identified by her very supportive Spirit Guide, Hector. This included several dark forces and many Earthbound spirits and soul fragments who were exceptionally fearful. Hector said that Sheila maintained a negative atmosphere around her that had to do with her future and then blurted out, "It's her excuses." Her Spirit Guide now informed me that he had two lifetimes with Sheila as her husband. They were hard lifetimes but happy ones, with many children. All foreign energy was removed successfully, no past lifetimes were found to contribute to her fears, and she has not been fragmented. Instructions on protection and powerful suggestions followed.

Sheila arrived for a second session eighteen months later, presenting with a fear of not being good enough, fear of hurting others, and a fear of doing the wrong thing. Her fear of driving had improved but not completely. I attempted to regress Sheila into a life, and when she was about to step into that life she screamed with fright and yelled out, "I'm in a box.... I'm in a box!"

This was followed by incessant crying until I told her, "You're now getting out of the box." She stopped crying as I immediately took her back to a life that she had with her Spirit Guide who was her husband in that lifetime. Once the patient was in that lifetime she began to relax and smile. Knowing that her Spirit Guide loves her and that he was excited about that life, I decided to call for him. Her Guide immediately came forward and was very willing to check Sheila for foreign energy. He let me know that she had forty-two dark force entities, including powerful ones, eight Earthbound spirits, and over 200 soul fragments. The exorcism required the help of all the Archangels, Master Spirits, St. Germain, and Jesus, in order to encapsulate and remove all forty-two dark force entities. Many of the Earthbound spirits were fearful of many things, and when I asked the rather large number of soul fragments to step forward if they had fears, almost all of them did so, according to the Spirit Guide. Once again we see Earthbound spirits and soul fragments being drawn to a host that they can identify with, one that has similar problems resulting from similar emotional trauma. All Earthbound spirits agreed to go to the Light and did so, and a soul retrieval was carried out for the over 200 soul fragments, so that they could rejoin their souls. The patient was found to be fragmented, and a second soul retrieval was carried out so Sheila could once again be a complete soul and less vulnerable to entity infestation. The patient was again instructed in God Light visualization and affirmation, and the session ended on a good note.

Sheila returned for a third session two months later with a resurgence of fear of not being good enough and not driving safely. Also, she was still afraid of moving on with her life. It became obvious that she was not utilizing her protective measures as consistently as she had promised. The reappearance of fears brought to mind that the Law of Attraction is applying to her but in a very negative way. Her fears had drawn entities with fears similar to those that she had when I had first seen her. Her Spirit Guide detected over forty Earthbound spirits and several hundred soul fragments who were saturated with these fears, which had been made much worse by the presence of a massive number of dark forces.

Sheila's Spirit Guide now began to speak. "Sheila is a beacon for drawing negative, fearful entities. By forgiving all who need forgiveness, she will become stronger and be able to uncap her creativity. She needs to take action and be fearless with judgment, to let out what's in, and enjoy the process. She needs to make decisions and know her decisions are good. One of her main lessons in this life is to be brave and bold." At that moment I began to feel that I'm missing something. I know the positive Law of Attraction is increased by not only having a positive attitude but also by being forgiving; however the patient had already forgiven herself and certain people on her previous appointments. This encouraged me to ask if there is anything or anybody else to be forgiven. She had no answer.

Following a successful exorcism, the patient became noticeably excited and exclaimed, "I know what the problem is! I needed to forgive those eight Earthbound spirits who had attached to me earlier for causing me problems, and I am now forgiving the many Earthbound spirits that are presently attached and bringing me more problems." The patient then forgave them from the bottom of her heart, and I assisted in helping them get to the Light. Following this, I returned the several hundred soul fragments to their original souls utilizing a massive soul retrieval.

When the patient all of a sudden had that insight, saying that she knew what the problem was, I thought to myself, "Once again, I am seeing evidence that the analytic and judgmental conscious mind is fully awake and functional while under deep hypnosis."

Sheila now began to smile, no longer bearing a fearful look. Her Guide found her to be fragmented and assisted me in doing a soul retrieval, making her once again a complete soul. I followed with powerful suggestions and again emphasized the importance of consistently carrying out her protective God Light visualizations and affirmations. The patient woke up extremely positive and happy and could not stop smiling. A follow up phone call eleven days later revealed that many of her fears have lessened considerably, and she is still smiling and feeling happy but not yet moving forward as much as she would like.

The patient returned two months later and told me that she was still smiling and definitely less afraid to move on with her life. She also informed me that she has been carrying out her God Light visualizations and affirmations to a much greater degree than she ever has. Many of her fears have diminished, but she still has an occasional panic reaction when driving, feeling that she may not be able to maneuver her car in time. When taken back to the cause of this problem, she saw herself as a baby, crying in the dark as her parents ferociously yelled at each other, and then saw herself at the age of three or four years old, feeling alone and helpless as the parental arguments continued. This was one of many frightening times in her childhood which induced confusion and panic, not knowing whether to run out of the room or stay put. As a result she usually remained frightened and afraid to move. Her Spirit Guide interrupted and insisted that the fear of maneuvering herself in these situations has carried over to her driving and many other areas of her life. Now that she understands why she felt the way she did, she will not feel the need to panic any more.

As the session continued, the Spirit Guide checked for foreign energy and found that she had no attached dark force entities, two Earthbound spirits who had just joined her, and one soul fragment who had fragmented from his soul due to a fear of driving. I was confident that the minimal amount of foreign energy that was discovered was due to her being more consistent with her protective measures. I was also gratified to hear from her Spirit Guide that she was a complete soul and has not been fragmented, as she has been in the past. I followed with an hypnotic balancing of her chakras, which I modified so as to make the patient feel younger, and gave further instructions in protective measures. The patient left smiling and said that she plans to uncap her creativity.

Eight months later Sheila came back for a reinforcement session. She said she still is smiling and feels good; however, she still has a slight fear of driving on freeways and also needs a boost in self-confidence. During her session I learned that she has carried out her protective measures faithfully and has been dating a "wonderful" man for four months. Also, she is excited over a granddaughter, who is due to deliver in the very near future and has a great desire to learn more about playing the piano. Sheila feels that she is definitely moving forward and is uncapping her creativity in a steady fashion.

Her Spirit Guide, Hector, came on board immediately during the session and informed us that Sheila has no foreign energy and has had a very small fragmentation of her own soul due to doubt. A soul retrieval was immediately accomplished, after which her Spirit Guide announced that he was proud of her accomplishments, and his advice to her is, "to live, trust, and be open to God's gifts."

ANGER MANAGEMENT

I have had many cases that clearly show how much influence soul fragments from another person's soul or consciousness can have upon the personality and actions of its host. One of these cases involved a patient by the name of Marvin, a 32-year-old man who was brought in by his wife, Brenda, who told me that her husband had become verbally abusive over the past several months and remained in a very angry mood.

Marvin turned out to be a good subject and easily entered deep hypnosis. His Spirit Guide was especially helpful and identified eight dark force entities and four soul fragments. Following a successful exorcism, the dark forces were totally removed. I now began interviewing the soul fragments which had attached to Marvin. It seems that each fragment had separated from its soul due to the emotional trauma of extreme anger and rage. One fragment came from a prostitute who was beaten instead of being paid by her customer. Another had to do with a gambler who bet and lost a small fortune in a poker game which he felt he could easily win. The third soul fragment was from a man who came home after work only to discover that two men had broken into his home, raped his wife, and beat his teenaged son. The fourth fragment had separated from the soul of an elderly man who, following his departure from a crowded subway, discovered that someone had stolen his wallet.

The patient's Spirit Guide said that all of these fragments had joined Marvin within the past six months and then ended the session by helping me carry out a soul retrieval, saying, "These exceptionally angry soul fragments have been returned to their respective souls; there is no further foreign energy. I feel that these fragments were mostly responsible for Marvin's aggressive behavior. He is not fragmented and will feel much calmer now. I send him Light and love." I followed with protective instructions.

I received a phone call from Brenda several months later, and she told me that Marvin was much improved and back to his old self.

THOUGHTS IN REGARD TO ENTITY POSSESSION

The ramifications of these uninvited infestations are beyond belief. In these situations we know that one's free will is being interfered with, and that a person is not completely culpable for creating his reality and truly can become a victim. Belief in spirit attachments is irrelevant since permission is not asked for nor given. Most of the time the host remains unaware of the attachment, especially if this attachment occurred when the host was a young child.

Enlightened individuals with a reasonable knowledge of the spirit world can also create their own vulnerability, which may occur during extreme emotional situations and under all the conditions that increase one's vulnerability. I believe that this vulnerability of individuals, with or without knowledge of spirit attachment, comes about without the host's intention, and therefore the responsibility for the host's actions must be shared with the spirit attachments.

A current attachment can cause unusual behavior patterns, personality changes, inappropriate speech or accents that may be noticed by the host or those close to the host. The medical community has many labels for these conditions, such as psychosis, schizophrenia, multiple personality disorder, and foreign accent syndrome to name a few. I feel very strongly that evaluation under deep hypnosis should be undertaken before a patient is given the stigma of a mental illness diagnosis.

The daily news is full of horrific incidents that carry the stench of evil. How true these words are, for within days of writing this I found myself hearing about the horrible residue from such evil acts while listening to the world news on February 27, 2012. At the time I was exercising and working up a good sweat. The radio announcer began talking about a high school student pulling a gun out in the school cafeteria and shooting several high school students in an Ohio town east of Cleveland. I began to become more interested when I heard "Ohio town, east of Cleveland," but when I heard the words "Chardon High School," I immediately stopped exercising and experienced an overwhelming feeling of personal involvement. Chardon, Ohio, was the town in which I practiced medicine for over thirty-two years. I thought to myself, "I probably delivered many of those high school students." I then felt a wave of panic flow through me as I remembered my one daughter still lives there, and her children probably go to that high school. Within minutes I put a call in to my daughter, but all I could do was leave a message. I turned on CNN and heard that one student was dead and four students were injured, two critically. I was not able to relax until my daughter finally called me with the news that my two grandchildren were okay. At that time she was trying to recover from the grueling anguish that she and other parents suffered through while waiting outside the school for news about their children. The school was under lockdown, and nobody could enter or leave or get information about who was shot. I later found out that both grandchildren were present in the school and that my fifteen-year-old grandson happened to have been in the classroom adjacent to the cafeteria where the shooting took place. The news soon reported that three students had been killed. Discussing this tragedy with my wife and having my family traumatized by the proximity to the killings, I had an overwhelming conviction that this teenage boy who committed this evil crime had to be saturated with dark forces.

We often wonder *what possessed* a person to be able to kill innocent people or children or execute thousands as the Nazis did in the years of World War II. The current craze involving suicide bombers is a sterling example of how dark forces are pursuing their evil agenda.

My research has shown that sometimes the psychological trauma involved when one becomes an organ donor precipitates a fragmentation of the donor's soul, and that fragment may follow the transplanted organ and attach to the organ recipient. Also, a deceased organ donor's Earthbound spirit may follow its organ and attach to the organ recipient. It is therefore a good idea to utilize protective measures prior to and following surgery involving the recipient of an organ transplant from a living or a deceased donor.

What I have presented here may well strike the reader as a "Get Out of Jail Free" card or the acceptance of the excuse, "The Devil made me do it." This is not my intention; however, my experience seems to indicate that attached entities of all sorts are able to exert a great influence on people's lives, the negative aspects of which are enhanced by the presence of dark forces which can be attached to the entities or to the host. When a large number of dark forces are present or if powerful dark forces are involved, the host can become unbelievably evil and capable of carrying out the most heinous of acts.

So what's the answer? What do we do with this information? Once again, the inimical monkey wrench has been thrown into the works and threatens to weaken our understanding of karma and reincarnation. Its devastating ripples can also spread to our legal system in the future and open the door to confusion and a treasure trove of useful information for defense attorneys. No longer will the plea of temporary insanity be needed; it would be replaced by the influence of entity attachment and point to the fact that the defendant was victimized and his free will was interfered with, resulting in his not being fully responsible for the crime. As I said before, the ramifications of these uninvited infestations are beyond belief. We would all agree that the world we live in is complicated enough and that the rule of law is necessary if we are to remain in a civilized world and avoid anarchy. Most people would not even consider or accept the concept of entity possession. Many people would think that the idea of past lifetimes affecting us was bad enough; but now they are being told that there are invisible entities that are attached to us and are also affecting us.

All I can say is what I've come across is real. The effects on the patient are very real. The communication to the entities through the patient is actually happening, and it's all coming from the patient's subconscious mind. Most importantly, the problems coming from an entity leave with the entity, and the patient is now free to live a life that he controls. The karmic monkey wrench is no longer there to interfere with his desires and his free will. If the patient keeps himself or herself protected and avoids situations that will increase his or her vulnerability, the protective status quo will remain, and the patient will have a much better opportunity to live a happy and healthy life.

Chapter 9

PAST LIFE INFLUENCE

AN EXTREME EMOTION CAN MANIFEST PHYSICALLY

Past life experiences would mean nothing if it were not for the sub-conscious mind, which can recall moment to moment details of every life we have lived, as well as every moment of the interim. These intricately detailed memories of one's life or the afterlife in between incarnations are filed away in an orderly fashion in the end-less reservoir of the subconscious mind which integrates these mem-ories and, as such, helps form our personality, our attitude, and our emotional feelings. The subconscious is our connection to the spiri-tual dimension, where time is conspicuously absent. When we leave the physical world by experiencing bodily death, our eternal soul or consciousness continues to carry on and carries with it our sub-conscious mind with its eternal memories. Thus emotional past life memories are able to surface and take on the afterlife quality of no distinction of time, which helps explain why a very emotional past life memory can affect our present life as much as it does. It's as if the memory had to do with something that just occurred. Thus the memory of an emotionally negative experience from a past lifetime that was brought to the forefront of the subconscious by something in the person's present life can have an extremely destructive effect. Such a memory is able to affect a person in this way by programming that person's conscious mind in a very negative way and causing that person to suffer and not have a clue why.

Fear is most often found to be the extreme emotion felt prior to a traumatic incident in a past life. This trauma may or may not have resulted in death. I have had cases where the predominant emotion in the past life was anger, which sometimes escalated to rage. These cases sometimes involved a present life situation wherein the patient manifested extreme anger followed by a physical condition that caused him to have chronic pain or a disfigurement related to a specific location on his body.

When I come across situations like this and ask the Spirit Guide to take the patient back to the cause of the patient's problem, the cause is often a past event which will clearly show that there was intense anger involved, and the traumatic injuries were located on the same areas of the patient's body that were involved in the patient's present-life incident. The patient's conscious mind will now observe what the subconscious brings forth, recognize the same emotions and feelings that he had during the present life event that brought on the pain or disfigurement, and finally understand how and why this traumatic past life memory affected him. The patient's conscious mind is now able to make a judgment and a distinction of time, thus enabling the patient to release the effect and improve his situation, often to the point where he is cured. This series of mental events will demonstrate to the patient how heightened emotions can become a prominent memory in the subconscious mind and how easily this emotional trauma can lead to a present day physical manifestation as a result of this memory from another time and another place. What we are talking about here is "cell memory."

My experience in carrying out thousands of Comprehensive Hypnoregressions has proven to me that every cell, and probably the most minute of sub-atomic particles in a person's body, retain the subconscious memory of every moment of every life that person has lived. These memories were filed away with a great diversity of emotions, which became an intrinsic part of the memory. Cell memory is a term used by several authors to describe the subconscious memory involved in causing a present-day physical illness, pain, or disfigurement. This cell memory is usually related to an injury or the way a person died in a past life, wherein the same area of the body that was involved in the past life injury or illness becomes the target for a present life illness, pain, or disfigurement, which can be initiated in the present life by a person from that past life, a strong emotion that was present at the time of the injury, or circumstances that were reminiscent of that extremely painful past life situation. These and possibly other causes can be responsible for setting off the recall of this very emotional memory in the subconscious mind and allowing it to stimulate cell memory and thus inflict physical discomfort and dysfunction. I prefer to call this cell memory "subconscious cell memory," which is easily accessible under deep hypnosis, a very therapeutic altered state of consciousness.

I feel that subconscious cell memory is also responsible for many organ transplant recipients reporting various changes in their attitude, personality, and preferences for food and entertainment, that were found to be very similar to that of the donor. Along the same lines, I had a patient who was a strapping construction worker who received a kidney from an older woman and within six months began to take up crocheting an afghan.

I have seen cases, such as Bell's Palsy, that were related to a subconscious memory of a traumatic past life incident that was bathed in anger and allowed to surface due to a present-day occurrence involving a similar degree of overwhelming anger. Subconscious cell memory helps explain many situations. Another case of great interest was presented by Paul Pearsall, Ph.D., a psychoneuroimmunologist. The case was about an eight-year-old girl who was murdered. Her heart was transplanted into a nine-year-old recipient who had vivid and lucid dreams about the murder, so much so that she was able to identify the assailant, who was then apprehended and brought to justice.

Exposing this very emotional cause of a patient's physical problem to the conscious mind under deep hypnosis is extremely helpful in improving the physical problem and is often curative. I have seen such cures occur immediately or over time; but when they don't, there may be other factors to be evaluated in a second appointment. For instance, is the patient carrying out his God Light visualizations and affirmations after his initial appointment when entities were removed in addition to identifying past life causes? If the patient is not keeping himself protected as much as possible he may be allowing entities to perpetuate his problem that was initiated by the recall of a traumatic emotional memory from a past life. As I have mentioned before, individuals with particular problems may act as a magnet to attract Earthbound souls or soul fragments with a similar situation. Also, dark forces always make things worse.

THE POWER OF FORGIVENESS

Why is it so important to forgive? If someone has hurt you, caused you to suffer, or made you miserable and unhappy, there is always a need to forgive. By not forgiving, you continue to wear the heavy chains of unforgivingness. If you continue to try to get even and want that person to be punished and even look forward to seeing him suffer, those chains will become heavier, and "the poisons of unforgivingness" that are generated will eventually cause you to become ill, emotionally and mentally at first, and later, physically.

Many people think that you are handing control over to the person you are forgiving. It's just the opposite. You are actually gaining control of the situation by forgiving the person, and you do this by actually saying the words and letting them come from within your heart. By doing so you will not only experience an unbelievable feeling of freedom and peace of mind as you free yourself from those chains of unforgivingness, you will also sense a feeling of health and happiness because you have now brought the law of attraction into play. A forgiving state of mind will truly become a magnet for attracting good things, and by putting positive words and thoughts out into the universe, especially words of forgiveness, you intuitively know the karmic return will be both positive and good.

It is vital to point out the power of forgiveness to patients. All too often I have come across patients who have been molested by their parents. When I explain that they have chosen their parents just as they have chosen all the varying aspects of their incarnation into this present life, they voice a rather emotional objection and often ask why they would have chosen such parents. My answer to these patients is, "You must learn to step back and look at the big picture. You chose your parents just as you have chosen everything that has to do with your incarnation into this world on Earth, all in the name of learning lessons... and just maybe one of those lessons was forgiveness."

BLACKNESS

There are some patients who have a distinct fear of hypnosis. When taken back to the cause of this fear, most of the patients go back to the moment of death during a past life and zero in on seeing just blackness once they experience that moment of death. This vivid and very emotional subconscious memory begins to associate seeing blackness with the death experience and this misinterpretation or misperception can easily spill over into the patient's present lifetime when an event triggers the activation of this very emotional subconscious memory. Patients with problems like this, and I have had many, often develop a fear of going to sleep, going under anesthesia, or undergoing hypnosis. This misbelief due to a misperception can easily be cured by convincing the patient to allow himself to be hypnotized and taking him back to the cause.

One could also speculate that in a past life the individual may have been buried alive because of inadequate assessment of death made during centuries when people were less educated in determining when a person has truly ceased to live. There have been cases of disinterment whereupon scratch marks were found on the inner roof of the casket. A past life memory related to this situation would definitely enhance the fear and worsen the phobia, especially if raw, terrifying emotions were experienced while waiting to die in cold, silent, suffocating blackness.

NEGATIVE PROGRAMMING FROM PAST LIVES, INCLUDING A FEAR OF DEATH

Of all of man's fears, fear of death is probably the most prevalent fear in the world today. This of course relates to a fear of the unknown and a fear of leaving those you love. I reiterate that the same description of life after death from millions of people who have experienced regression and from those who have undergone near death experiences gives us a pretty good idea of what to expect when we take that inevitable journey into the unknown.

The case in point is about Edith, a 41-year-old woman from Great Britain who voiced this fear and in addition was deathly afraid of being cremated. She also was quite impatient and sarcastic and allowed her temper to flare all too often.

Following induction, Edith proved to be a good subject, and her Spirit Guide was exceptionally helpful and after thoroughly checking for the frequencies of foreign energy pronounced Edith free of foreign energy with no fragmentation of her soul. When I asked Edith's Spirit Guide to take her back to the cause of her fear of cremation, she went back to a past life where she attempted to save her mother from a fire on the second floor of their home. Edith was very concerned that she would also die in that smoldering inferno while trying to save her mother. Edith did not die in that fire, but her mother did. This fear-laden emotional memory has remained prominent in her subconscious and has been responsible for negatively programming her conscious mind whenever she sees, hears, or experiences fire in any way.

When I asked her Spirit Guide to go back to the cause of the patient's short temper and sarcasm, we visited three past lifetimes.

The first had to do with a life in the days of the flourishing Roman Empire. In that lifetime Edith was a Roman general who could only get the cooperation of his soldiers by shouting and becoming extremely angry. The second lifetime took place in ancient China, where Edith was a teacher of rebellious and rowdy children. In that lifetime, shouting and becoming quite angry was a necessary element when teaching students who didn't listen. The third lifetime found the patient living in ancient Persia, where she had the responsibility of teaching the skill of weaving to pitifully ignorant women. This hopeless plight brought out much in the way of sarcasm and anger in Edith during that lifetime.

In a follow up visit several months later the patient reported that her fear of death and being cremated was definitely diminished, and she was much less sarcastic, much more patient, and no longer harbored a short fuse as far as her temper was concerned. She now wanted me to work on the fact that she eats more when under stress. When I addressed this issue with her Spirit Guide, he immediately took us to an event that occurred during the American Civil War. In that lifetime Edith was a Confederate soldier by the name of Jesse who had become separated from his unit and was running as fast as he could in the fields, knowing that Yankee soldiers were not far behind. He was extremely scared, tired, and hungry when he stumbled upon an abandoned home in the woods. He entered the house and discovered lots of food, which he ate to the point of vomiting and having abdominal pain. He wrapped up the remaining food and took it with him as he continued to run. Soon he came upon another group of Southerners on the run and joined them. This made him feel safer, especially since they had food. The group traveled for quite a distance and was eventually taken in by a plantation owner, whom they helped by doing chores. The war ended. Jesse remained at that plantation and had definitely gained excessive weight by continuing to eat when under stress.

Edith could now clearly see that the lifetime that occurred during the strife of the Civil War was a definite cause of her eating unnecessarily whenever she is stressed. A follow up visit many months later showed the patient to be improved on all her issues, including emotional eating. Also her Spirit Guide informed me that the patient is a Light Worker and is able to ward off uninvited foreign energy.

QUIETLY LIVING ALONE

I would like to mention that I have seen two patients who manifested living habits that were characteristic of the way monks lived hundreds of years ago. When taken back to the cause of these situations they regressed to a life as a Tibetan monk, which explained why they preferred to quietly live alone. They often had a great affinity for old books, candles, paper, and ink. When their Spirit Guide was asked to show the patients their blueprint that they had designed for themselves in that lifetime, they were able to observe and understand why they lived as they did. The lessons that these patients were to learn in that life were almost identical. They were: you only need to learn and to think; you don't require material goods; everything you'll ever need is in your hands; and finally, it is not necessary for you to speak, rather just write things down.

SHEDDING UNBELIEVABLE LIMITATIONS

A good example of such limitations has to do with a prior lifetime that caused a devastating influence on Samantha, a 29-year-old woman from a small town in Texas. It seems that she could never comfortably carry on a conversation with a stranger, someone she had never met. If she found herself in a situation where she had to speak with someone she didn't know, she would experience a panic reaction wherein she would tremble, stutter, perspire profusely and become nauseated. Physicians gave her various medications for the problem but could not help her, and so she remained very limited personally, professionally, and especially socially.

Under deep hypnosis, Samantha's Spirit Guide helped me uncover the cause of her problem by taking her back to a past life as Victoria in 18th century England. She was born into royalty, and by age seven had become a social butterfly, so much so that she socialized with everyone, even commoners. One fateful day two young men approached her and her trainer during riding lessons and said they wanted to show her a beautiful horse that she might ask her parents to buy. They said the horse was just outside the gate to her parents' property. Victoria's trainer objected, but Victoria socialized with the young men and happily agreed to ride over to see the horse. Once Victoria and her trainer were outside the gate, the two men became extremely violent and subdued Victoria and her trainer. Leaving the trainer tied to a tree with a note, the two men brought out their two horses and rode off with Victoria.

Victoria's parents were quite upset when they read the note left with the trainer; it demanded a small fortune for Victoria's return. According to Samantha's Spirit Guide, the two men were not aware of how powerful Victoria's father was. Within one day and by that evening, the two kidnappers were apprehended and Victoria was returned to her father, who sternly waved his finger at her and shouted, "From this day forward, you will never speak to strangers!"

This very emotional memory was imprinted so deeply into Samantha's subconscious mind that when a stranger addresses her, or she is introduced to someone she has never met, this very emotional past life memory is ignited and brought to the forefront of her subconscious mind, where it is able to program her conscious mind in a devastating way and prevent her from being comfortably able to speak. Under hypnosis she was able to make a distinction of time, namely that this happened a long time ago; thus she was now able to understand that this powerful memory was responsible for a misbelief based on a misperception, and as a result, she is now able to fully release the negative programming of her conscious mind and put an end to her suffering.

Within a matter of days Samantha felt as if she had been reborn. She no longer holds back from meeting new people and no longer panics when she does meet them. She and her family are now experiencing much more joy and happiness in their lives. I've had other cases similar to this with much the same outcome.

THE POWERFUL INFLUENCE OF PAST LIFE EVENTS

The following case clearly shows how very emotional events in one's past lifetimes can create or contribute to several emotional and physical problems in that person's present life. Phyllis was a 55-year-old woman from Utah who came to see me so as to improve the state of several emotional and physical maladies that have plagued her for years. These included depression, hypertension, macular degeneration, migraine headaches, and a vague discomfort in her stomach.

Phyllis easily slipped into a deep hypnotic state, and almost immediately I had a very helpful Spirit Guide on board who said he had been her Guide for many lifetimes. Phyllis exhibited no foreign energy whatsoever and had not been fragmented; and when taken back to the cause of her depression she saw herself as a male medic for the Confederate army during the Civil War who was very beaten down over the disabling injuries and senseless loss of so many lives. Her Spirit Guide said this was one of four lifetimes that were responsible for her depression.

A lifetime in Austria in the 1800s saw her as a young woman who lost many loved ones during the plague. In the early 1900s she was a 19-year-old woman in Ireland who witnessed lots of fighting and suffering amongst the Irish and the English. Senseless killing continued because of religion. The patient in that lifetime died at 19 years old when a horse ran over her during the fighting. Phyllis' present lifetime also contributed to her depression due to a trying childhood on her parents' farm. Her parents argued constantly, and she felt that her father never liked her.

When taken back to the cause of her hypertension, Phyllis once again saw herself as the Confederate medic during the Civil War with the impossible task of trying to care for the many wounded men during the battles. The Spirit Guide said that the suffering she underwent in Ireland also contributed as did her present lifetime, mostly because her sister constantly manipulated her. According to Phyllis' Spirit Guide her macular degeneration was also related to that lifetime during the Civil War. As a medic, he was constantly exposed to the smoke from the gunfire, which continued to injure his eyes.

The cause of the migraine headaches was related to the way she died during the upheaval in Ireland. A horse ran her over, and the horse's hoof kicking her head is what killed her. The Guide also said that there was a genetic disposition in her present life that helped initiate migraine headaches.

When taken back to the source of her stomach problems, she again revisited her days as a medic in the Civil War and immediately saw that there was a tremendous lack of food, and when he was able to find food, it was bad. A second lifetime in ancient Rome as a Roman officer in charge of many soldiers also contributed to the stomach problems which resulted from the stress from the political upheaval of the day.

Forgiveness of herself and of prominent people in her present life that have hurt her in one way or another was carried out, thus releasing Phyllis from the chains of unforgivingness. Following this, I attempted to have her understand that these past lifetimes have greatly influenced her present lifetime in a negative way, since negative programming of the conscious mind had now been put in motion by her subconscious mind following the resurfacing of prominent memories that were filed away in those past lifetimes with exceptionally powerful negative emotions. The trigger that allowed these subconscious memories to surface could have been a person from that life or an event or situation that was reminiscent of one in that lifetime. Sometimes even a sound or smell could trigger such memories. Whatever the reason for bringing up these memories subconsciously, the effect is the same, namely negative programming of the conscious mind by the subconscious, causing the person to suffer without consciously knowing why.

I explained to Phyllis that once she was able to understand that the events in those past lifetimes were responsible for her emotional and physical problems, and once she was able to understand that they occurred a long time ago and do not affect or relate to her present life, she should easily be able to release the effect. I followed with powerful suggestions and protective measures to her subconscious mind, namely to carry out God Light visualizations and affirmations routinely.

Several weeks later a follow up call revealed that the patient was feeling much better. The migraine headaches were gone, and all of her physical and emotional problems were improved. Two years later a follow up call revealed that the patient still feels great and that none of her presenting issues have returned except for very occasional migraine headaches.

MORE SUFFERING FROM NEGATIVE PROGRAMMING

Another example of an emotional past life memory causing great suffering is a case involving a fifty-five year-old man who had low back pain for many years. The back pain was diagnosed many years ago as a manifestation of multiple sclerosis. Under deep hypnosis, an Earthbound spirit that had died at 82 years old was discovered. This Earthbound spirit had frequent arthritic back pain in his life. According to the patient's Spirit Guide, this Earthbound spirit contributed to the patient's back pain; however, the main cause of this pain was from a traumatic past life memory that had subconsciously surfaced and was programming the patient's conscious mind in a very negative way.

When taken back to the cause of his back pain emanating from his multiple sclerosis, this patient regressed to the early 16th century as a ten-year-old boy who found himself near a battle scene witnessing much turmoil, fire, and screaming throughout a village as horsemen rode through it. An explosion occurred very close to him and threw him a distance, making him dizzy. He was unable to stand but found he could crawl and make his way to a cave, where he took refuge. His spine and low back caused him great pain.

The patient's Spirit Guide then showed us the event in his present life that caused the subconscious memory to surface. It occurred when the patient was five years old. Living in a foster home at that time, he fell and injured his hip. He couldn't tell anybody about his injury because he was afraid they would send him away. The patient's conscious mind was now putting all this information together, and when the patient awoke from hypnosis, he felt a sense of peace and understanding come over him. Follow up eight months later revealed that the patient had left the session without the back pain, and the pain has still not returned.

PAST LIFE CONNECTION TO ALCATRAZ

One of my most interesting cases involving a past life influence had to do with a nine-year-old girl who was diagnosed with Attention Deficit Hyperactivity Disorder (ADHD). This young lady was becoming progressively more hostile with her sibling and often spoke of hurting herself and others. She was becoming more compulsive and her aggressive attitude was becoming a definite problem in school in spite of her being on several medications. On several occasions after she had gotten into trouble she would say, "I wish I could just die."

Following hypnotic induction I was able to communicate with her Spirit Guide. I asked her Spirit Guide why this young patient was so hyperactive and giving the impression that she would like to hurt herself and others. At that moment the patient began to see herself as a 20-year-old male prisoner in Alcatraz. The prisoner's name in that lifetime was Marques. He said he was convicted of murdering an individual by the name of Jacob, following an altercation. I asked the Guide if Marques had dark forces attached to him. The Guide said yes, and that five of those same dark forces are presently attached to the patient as well. Following this revelation I conducted an exorcism and removed the dark forces. The Guide then confirmed that her soul was complete, with no other foreign energy present. I then stressed the importance of the God Light visualization and affirmation.

During a follow up call several months later, I was told by the parents that there definitely was some improvement, fewer outbursts, no further "meltdowns" in school, and a tendency to be more courteous. The parents informed me that they had located the Alcatraz archives which listed Armand Marques as Inmate #69. The parents also said that when their daughter was six years old, she was taught how to go online and look up things. The first thing that came to this six-year-old's mind was to look up Alcatraz.

CHOOSING TO BE A DARK FORCE ENTITY

Gloria was a forty-eight-year-old, extremely intelligent and talented woman from Wisconsin who presented with long-term depression, in addition to a lack of self-worth, panic attacks, insomnia, claustrophobia, and a knowing that there is an obstruction to her moving forward in life. Her history revealed frequent molestation in her early teens by a family member, a variety of addictions which she has conquered, and many alien abductions. Following induction the patient attained deep hypnosis, and her Spirit Guide, Mark, came forth immediately after being summoned. Five dark forces, including powerful ones, were removed. The remaining foreign energy consisted of a great many extraterrestrials, which included both benevolent Reptilians and demonic Grays.

According to her Spirit Guide, the patient was a Light Worker, and in her last life she was the leader of benevolent Reptilians on their own planet. One of the benevolent Reptilians was attached to her, and the remaining multitude hovered nearby. Their purpose in being here was to guard and protect her. The demonic Grays, however, were trying to control her but were unable to, due to the excessive amount of Light within her. They joined her when she was four years old and abducted her many times, during which they did mind experiments and removed one egg, which was never fertilized. Upon being discovered, the demonic Grays left, and no implants remained. Gloria's Spirit Guide felt that all the benevolent Reptilians should be allowed to stay with her.

Gloria's soul had undergone an unbelievable amount of trauma in her present life, and thus her soul was found to be extremely fragmented. An extensive soul retrieval was carried out, allowing Gloria to once again be a complete soul. Protective suggestions followed.

Gloria's Spirit Guide, Mark, now began to reveal the fact that Gloria had a life in Atlantis as an evil queen, a very dark life. At this moment I had to take a deep breath because I couldn't believe what I was hearing. The Spirit Guide then said that Gloria also had evil lifetimes in Africa and during the Mayan era. Here I was, hearing from a very valid Spirit Guide that a Light Worker chose to be evil in several lifetimes. I thought to myself, "This is a contradiction in terms!" Shaking off the effect of this most recent surprise, I led the patient into understanding that it is important that she forgive herself for choosing those evil lifetimes. The forgiveness came forth from deep within her heart.

We then uncovered the fact that the obstruction to moving forward in life was from her fear of unworthiness, which was being self-created and stemmed from living those evil lives. Of course, this was enhanced and made much worse by attached dark forces.

When Gloria was taken back to the cause of her claustrophobia, her subconscious mind recalled a past life in Africa, where she displeased her husband, who had many wives. As a punishment she was buried alive in a tomb and died a cruel death of suffocation. Before the session ended the patient's Spirit Guide, Mark, said that this is Gloria's last life on Earth and in this dimension.

The patient returned six weeks later for a second session, saying that the first session helped her for a few days and then sadness and depression took over. The induction went well, and her Spirit Guide came on the scene almost immediately, saying he invited a Master Spirit by the name of Fohat to join us, so he may clarify and help with Gloria's healing. Within seconds Master Spirit Fohat was present and saying, "It is important that you know that Gloria is also a Master Spirit. She still is without foreign energy, but her soul fragmented again when she found out that she chose evil lifetimes. It is imperative that she understand that as a Master Spirit she chose these evil lifetimes with good reason, namely to understand the duality of good versus evil, so she will know better how to defeat the dark forces. As a dark force, she did not do very bad things." The session ended following a second soul retrieval on the patient and a reminder for her to be persistent in carrying out her protective measures.

The next day I received an email from Gloria, and the subject title was, "A very great afternoon!" The first line of the email read, "I can't seem to get this smile off my face, and this time, after yesterday, I know it will last!" The entire theme of the email was gratitude. It ended with, "The Light of God never fails."

In the same vein I have had a few more patients also presenting with a host of problems which I found to be related to not only past lifetimes but to a bizarre life-changing decision made by their souls during or between their many lifetimes. One of those patients also chose to be a dark force entity so as to learn, to grow, and to discover what evil is, so she would understand what is truly good–in other words, for reasons that are not basically evil. Master Spirits were intervening and influencing the decisions that these patients were making, a situation that I have not encountered in my research except for the case of primitive man, whose choices regarding incarnation were made by Master Spirits because this form of early man had not yet learned the lesson of love. As extraterrestrials, these patients were mostly without emotion, especially compassion, but during certain Earth lifetimes they displayed it and paid the price, namely that of excruciating guilt. They were learning the lesson of love just as primitive man did, namely that love cannot be belittled or eliminated from one's life, the obvious agenda of the dark forces. Loving and being kind is what it's all about.

THE POWER OF A PROMINENT PAST LIFE

Gregory is a fifty-nine-year-old college professor from Montana who presented me with a long list of issues, namely depression, inability to concentrate, feelings of unworthiness, anxiety, difficulty making decisions, procrastination, and being drawn to things that can cause problems and produce anxiety.

Under deep hypnosis the patient's Spirit Guide confirmed that there was no foreign energy present and that there has been no fragmentation of his soul. I now decided to ask the Spirit Guide to take the patient back to the cause of his procrastination. Within a few seconds the patient found himself in a medieval lifetime with two children who he recognized as his present children. The father and his two children had been walking along a mountain trail and were now trying to return home. When they came to a fork in the trail, the father was forced to make a decision and pick the right path that would take them home. As it turned out, he made the wrong decision and chose a trail that was very treacherous, so much so that his son had an accident causing him to never be able to walk again.

The patient in that lifetime blamed himself for being the cause of his son's injury and at the same time resented the heavy burden of caring for his crippled son. At this moment this very intuitive Spirit Guide carried on with a rather sterling explanation of how and why the patient felt as he did in his present lifetime. The Spirit Guide began by saying, "This very prominent past lifetime has been responsible for feelings of resentment and guilt toward Gregory's present son and for the procrastination that the patient displays in doing things, especially in making decisions, because he doesn't trust himself to make the right decision. It also has contributed to his being a perfectionist, mostly because he doesn't want to be wrong, and in the process has caused him to have a negative approach to life, always focusing on what can go wrong. This all added up to increased anxiety and a feeling of unworthiness. Such feelings have stayed with him through many lifetimes, keeping him anxious and unable to relax. This was also true in his present childhood. Many lifetimes with such feelings have resulted in a distrust of people and a fear of rejection. Thus Gregory has developed a problem understanding people's motives and has become fearful that they will hurt his feelings.

"Gregory enjoyed past lifetimes where he was quite rich. This had nothing to do with having a fortune; rather, it was because of having very little contact with people. He felt safer because he did not have to deal with friends or people at work, just servants. One of his happiest lifetimes was as a hermit with no outside contact. Yes, such lifetimes were safer, but because he did not do anything for anybody, these lifetimes subconsciously caused him to feel guilty and build up negative karma. One of his lessons was therefore to try to fix this by being around people and making up for lifetimes where he had been selfish.

"The weight of these massive feelings has overwhelmed Gregory to the point where he has been unable to concentrate and has resulted in depression, which has been increased by his empathy for others. Gregory didn't seem to realize that his lack of trust for people stemmed from the pain that his empathy for others brought him."

At this time I engaged in a lengthy dissertation on forgiving yourself and planted powerful suggestions in Gregory's subconscious mind regarding anxiety, procrastination, decision making, depression, concentration, self-confidence and self-esteem. Gregory's Spirit Guide then commented, "Gregory's lessons included the fact that he needs to lighten up and enjoy other people without taking responsibility for their feelings. He will do fine." At that moment I recalled that Gregory had said his present teenage son was depressed, hostile, and argumentative. Knowing the complicated relationship that his son had with Gregory in that lifetime, I thought that a remote entity releasement would be helpful for Gregory's son and decided to ask Gregory's Spirit Guide what he thought about this. The Spirit Guide agreed. I then closed with powerful suggestions to the patient about carrying out God Light visualizations and affirmations. Following the session we checked with Gregory's son about scheduling him for a remote entity releasement with my assistant so as to help him overcome his diminished self-worth, anger, depression and sadness.

I received a follow up on our session a few weeks later and was pleased to hear that Gregory had improved in all the issues that he presented with, and he was looking forward to being present at the remote session that would occur shortly to de-possess his son.

I received another call from Gregory a few months later, which included a follow up on his son's remote entity releasement, a session with his daughter who I saw within this same period, and himself. Gregory said his son is more cheerful, and they are communicating much better. His daughter is very much improved regarding the problems that were causing her much distress, and as far as he is concerned, Gregory still feels that the positive changes he has undergone are truly noteworthy.

PULLING OFF A CURE

Doing something over and over is a good definition of a habit. How do they begin? Why do they persist? Where do they come from? Good questions. Many times habits are developed in one's present lifetime. Hypnotic suggestions are very helpful here; however, some of the answers to those questions are in the subconscious mind. The habit may also be due to an attached entity who has transferred this repetitive action to its host, or it may be from a past life. In these cases, standard hypnotherapy can be helpful but usually won't stop the habit. It's important to take the patient back to the cause, expose it to the conscious mind, and do what's necessary to fully eliminate it, namely, have the patient gain a full understanding of the situation, possibly employ forgiveness of self and others, and utilize powerful suggestions to put a stop to the habitual action. The following case is an excellent example of this type of habit.

The condition of trichotillomania involves a neurotic habit which causes a person to pull his own hair. The hair may often be broken off in different lengths. This habit usually appears in early childhood and may remain undiagnosed for a long period of time. I saw such a patient several years ago. His father called me from Northern California and told me that his eighteen-year-old son, Kevin, has a hair-pulling problem that started when he was very young and has persisted in spite of various therapeutic regimens, some of which have been helpful but not curative, namely neuro-feedback and hypnosis. Kevin's father also informed me that the hair pulling worsens when Kevin becomes anxious. My response was, "If I can get to the cause of his problem under deep hypnosis, I am sure that he will improve."

Kevin easily slipped into a deep trance, and a valid Spirit Guide came through. The Guide was his true Spirit Guide but was not very confident or sure of the various forms of foreign energy he was identifying. I called for and was successful in getting a second, more experienced Spirit Guide to come forth and help. Following the successful exorcism of two dark forces I interrogated an Earthbound spirit and a soul fragment but was unable to uncover an entity responsible for Kevin's hair-pulling habit. The Spirit Guide made me aware of the fact that Kevin was an incomplete soul due to a traumatic incident which caused his soul to fragment. A successful soul retrieval was carried out, allowing Kevin to once again be a complete soul and less vulnerable to entity attachment.

At this point in the session I asked the two Spirit Guides to please take Kevin back to the cause of his hair-pulling habit. Kevin immediately found himself in a small, dark room, which he described as a medieval prison. He was a woman in her early twenties at this time, who had been caught and imprisoned for stealing food. Kevin could easily feel himself in this woman's body, pacing back and forth and fidgeting with her hair. She would wrap her long, brown hair along her fingers and drag her hand through her hair, occasionally pulling some hair out. An overview of that lifetime found this woman being treated in a cruel fashion and fed very little food, so that within two long, lonely years she died, and at the time of her death, she had very little hair on her head.

The remainder of the session was filled with forgiveness of the prison guards in that life and powerful suggestions to the subconscious to not touch his hair, but if he did, to reverse the position of his hand so that he would be touching his hair with the back of his hand and enjoying the comfortable sensations of his soft, smooth hair on the back of his hand. All of this will eventually lead him to become calmer and be pleased that his hair is looking great.

A follow up call two months later to his father revealed the fact that Kevin was doing quite well. His father said that he was very pleased to tell me that Kevin has not pulled his hair since the appointment.

TWO TYPES OF A DOUBLE WHAMMY

People are often exposed to both the influence of past lifetimes and that of entity possession. When this occurs, and interferes with something that is extremely important to that person, it can be devastating. Such was the case with Jack, a 28-year-old man from South Carolina who came to me with relationship problems. It seems that his girlfriend, Sherry, is a beautiful girl that he fell in love with during his youth. The feelings for each other were mutual but were being interfered with by his 'wandering eye,' as Sherry puts it. Jack has a problem focusing on his girlfriend when other women are nearby. The other problem is that Sherry's family does not think Jack is good enough for her and has subsequently discouraged any plans they have for marriage.

The hypnotic induction went well, and we were immediately able to communicate with a valid Spirit Guide who identified several Earthbound spirits, one of whom was a young male spirit who has been with Jack for many years. This Earthbound spirit loved to be distracted by women and has enjoyed bringing this trait to his host, Jack. At this point in the session, Jack's very helpful Spirit Guide said that Jack and Sherry had three lives together before their present lifetime. It turns out that they were lovers in two of those lives but could not marry because of family interference and as a result were extremely unhappy in those lifetimes.

Past lifetimes, such as Jack and Sherry had together, let them know that their present problems are not always new. Seeing the results of family interference in previous lifetimes should certainly reinforce this couple's dedication to each other so that they are free to spend their lives together as husband and wife. The Earthbound spirits, including the one who loved to be distracted by women, were sent to the Light, so I am sure that Jack's wandering eye problem will rapidly improve.

❦

Another form of dual interference in one's life can occur when a powerful past life influence originates from the same highly emotional memory, which is buried deep in the subconscious mind of the patient and in the subconscious mind of an attached Earthbound spirit. Some time ago I conducted an entity releasement on George, a depressed patient with even more of a double whammy situation, wherein the patient was consciously suffering because of the subconscious recall of an extremely sad past life memory from a life he had over two hundred years ago. In that lifetime George was forced to leave his family and join his country's army, which was defending the country from an invasion by an adjacent country which had a vicious and ambitious dictator who wanted to take over and control as much territory as he could. In that lifetime George found himself in a battle which was over a day's ride from his home. Hearing that the enemy broke through the defenses near his village, he left the battle scene and rode his horse all night to get home. Upon arriving at his village, George bore witness to the carnage the enemy left behind, including the mangled bodies of his wife and children. The trauma of their death caused their souls to stay together in the lower astral plane and not go to the Light. Eventually the souls of his wife and children were able to find and attach to George, where they felt more secure and together.

As Earthbound spirits, George's wife and children had a profound influence upon him, namely allowing their feelings of having been left alone, unprotected, and brutally murdered permeate George's feelings, which then triggered his own recall of this unthinkable and emotionally sad subconscious memory, which was also laden with guilt because he was not there for his family when they needed him. Thus his conscious mind was being brutally and almost constantly bombarded with this unmitigated sadness from a past life memory recall of a lamentable and cruel wartime occurrence, all of which has resulted in deep depression.

I was able to remove many dark forces and help George's Earthbound spirit family get to the Light, after which we wished them Godspeed. A soul retrieval was performed on George's fragmented soul. Several months later I was told that the patient has become much more tranquil but was to stay on his medication per his physician.

MY THOUGHTS ON ABANDONMENT

Every so often I encounter a patient with issues that are related to feelings of abandonment. Rather than going into the particulars of these cases, I would like to lay out my plan of attack. Following induction and deepening and taking the patient up to his Higher Self, I have the patient call forth a Spirit Guide who I will test to assure myself of his or her validity. I then check to see if any foreign energy is present and to see if there is any influence from attached entities who may be bringing about these issues which may be related to their own abandonment memories. Following interrogation and proper confirmed removal of all attached entities, I ask the Spirit Guide to take the patient to the cause of his feeling of abandonment. I then ask if any lifetimes initiated this feeling or contributed to it. There can be many reasons why a person feels abandoned, but if the cause is not clear, I have the Spirit Guide take the patient back in time in his present life to childhood and finally, to his intrauterine fetal life within his mother. I then take the patient through the birth process. During the prenatal stage and delivery, the attitudes and feelings of the parents, physicians, nurses, relatives, and friends are being picked up by the subconscious mind of the fetus and later, that of the newborn. If their comments are very negative, they can become prominent subconscious memories in the infant. More of this may occur during delivery if heavy sedation or general anesthesia is used. Under these circumstances, the mother's conscious mind is shut down and the bonding connection between the mother and newborn is interfered with. In the same way, if the infant is separated from his mother immediately following delivery for a significant period of time, the infant may be recording feelings of abandonment which may also cause problems downstream. These revelations will help the patient understand that birth trauma and feelings of abandonment due to these situations are common during the birthing experience. Once therapists carry out Comprehensive Hypnoregression and explore the subconscious with the patient, these feelings will be understood and released.

If a patient is still complaining of problems stemming from the feeling of abandonment, the therapist is obligated to also regress the patient back to the moment he was created by the Source, our

Creator, who is absolute perfection and the consciousness of All That Is. Our Creator, that which has been called God, created many souls in order to manifest, so He may experience and explore Himself in all dimensions. Each soul carries a spark of the Creator and has its own unique vibration. When the soul was part of God, it was part of His perfection. Once it was created it became imperfect with a need to return to its perfect state so it could eventually rejoin the Creator and again become an essential part of the Oneness of God.

Once the patient has regressed to the moment of his creation, the therapist should then regress him to the moment before his creation. The patient will now find himself in unbelievable bliss as he feels himself become an integral part of his Creator. The therapist will wait a few minutes while the patient enjoys this moment and then advance him once again to the moment that he was created. Following this, the therapist will explain to the patient that God did not abandon him. This was all a part of God's plan. If the patient's feeling of abandonment originated from his leaving the Creator and becoming an individual soul, it will now be released as the patient begins to fully understand that he was created for a purpose and not abandoned.

OBSTETRICS, THE NOBLE PROFESSION

All this talk about fetuses, birth, and newborns has awakened the obstetrician in me and brought forth memorable moments in my practice that flash on and off in my conscious mind. All the experience that I encountered in delivering close to 5,000 babies has not only enabled me to relate to and be a part of this very emotional time in a woman's life, it has also given me the opportunity to identify with the mother and father during the entire pregnancy and delivery. Fortunately the parents are usually not aware of the dangers involved from the myriad of complications of pregnancy and delivery; however, the obstetrician is, and some days it shows.

I would be willing to bet that most obstetricians choose this gut-wrenching, lack-of-sleep specialty on the very day that they delivered their first baby in training. In a way, I did, too, for this confirmed that not only was I meant to do this, to prevent problems such as brain damage, which can be devastating to the baby and the entire family, but also it allowed me to be able to take part in this joyous and miraculous occasion to assist our Creator and safely bring a new life into this world. Whether it's his first or his last delivery, an obstetrician will always harbor a great sense of pride and gratitude for such a privilege. Sometimes that joy is tempered with rampant emotions involving concern. The obstetrician somehow learns to quiet these feelings so he can function at peak efficiency and at the same time always remember that he is responsible for two lives.

Most people have no idea what situations obstetricians face during their many years in practice. These situations include managing complicated labor and delivery cases, twins, triplets, abnormal delivery presentations, fetal distress, patients in shock, emergency Caesarian sections, and ruptured tubal pregnancies, to name a few. Throw in complicated gynecological cases and performing major surgery on morbidly obese patients, and people begin to understand the challenges of this specialty.

Obstetricians cannot help but be compassionate, especially in regard to the two lives for which they are responsible, the mother and her child. Compassion has to be present in order for one to choose this specialty, which is full of stress, dangers, and sleepless nights, all of which seem to be negated when you experience the feeling of elation that penetrates your very being upon safely delivering a baby. As far as I am concerned, there is no feeling in the world that comes close. I truly believe that I am being of assistance to our Creator when I help bring a new life into the world. I must say that such a feeling has not diminished even after thousands of deliveries. I truly miss the experience but not the stress nor the moments when I had to tell a mother that the baby I just delivered was stillborn. I can still feel the empathy that permeated my mind and heart as the joyful excitement of the mother's face became shriveled and submersed in tears. All in all, my specialty had brought me closer to my Creator and taught me many lessons about life, some of which I could not explain until I found myself becoming spiritually enlightened.

PAST LIFE PERSONALITIES

Performing past life regression sessions has given me the opportunity to observe these lifetimes from afar, and this experience has shown me that people's personalities are truly the sum total of all their previous personalities. I believe the influence of a particular life can easily be seen when one observes the interactions that the patient has with people in his present life and especially with those in his family.

Sometimes the person's past life personality is extremely strong, and as such, it breaks through the time barrier and finds itself in the person's present lifetime. The arrival of the past life personality usually requires a rather strong stimulus for this to occur, one that is emotionally powerful. It may be related to excessive drug usage or extreme emotions such as rage, which may or may not be associated with traumatic circumstances. Such personalities may not fit or be appropriate for the present time.

When diagnosed with multiple personality disorders and the patient is undergoing further diagnostic investigation, Comprehensive Hypnoregression Therapy should be used. In doing so, the therapist would be able to make use of the patient's Spirit Guide and easily rule out an attached entity as the source of the personality and determine if a past life personality has come through. I believe that the answers to most of our problems lie in the subconscious mind, not in the conscious mind. I further theorize that if a person's traumatic situation is beyond his ability to cope with it, the subconscious mind may allow a stronger past life personality to reveal itself, take the place of the present personality, and handle the current problems.

Chapter 10

FUTURE LIFE INFLUENCE

Many years ago when I first began regressing patients back to the causes of their issues, I would sometimes just say, "Go to a life that explains the cause of your issue." Well, the patients did just that; however, some of the patients progressed to a future life. The case that follows was one of several cases that I have seen through the years and is understandable when one considers that time is a construct of the physical plane and does not exist in the spiritual dimension; thus a patient can be taken to a future life. I feel that this future life progression is actually a potential life, if one decides to choose it and live it; however, I may be wrong.

AHEAD OF HIS TIME

I reiterate that I never tire of surprises, and yes, they occur quite often. I am accustomed to past lifetimes influencing people in many ways, but the following case really bowled me over when I heard the patient's Spirit Guide explain that this patient's intelligence, as well as his proficiency at his extremely complex job in Great Britain, were both handed down to him from a future life.

When I asked the Spirit Guide to take us forward to that lifetime, this young patient found himself in an office building in a major city in the year 2060. At that time he was a young male architect doing industrial design work, primarily on vehicles and buildings. During my conversation with him in that lifetime, he spoke of having vehicles with an energy power source and the fact that these vehicles required no fuel.

What makes this case even more significant is the fact that this patient's present life consists of a high school education with no training whatsoever in physics, yet his prestigious job has him carrying out complex projects which require a knowledge of advanced physics and industrial design that other individuals are unable to handle. He added that he has always come through when pressure at work was excessive during very complex projects.

FUTURE LIFE ON ANOTHER PLANET

I have come across many patients who, under deep hypnosis, have described lifetimes on other planets as well as on Earth, and I have had patients who felt that they did not belong here on Earth, or discovered, under hypnosis, that this was their first life on Earth. I have also observed different patients being consistent in their description of a particular planet, its inhabitants, and the conditions that exist there during a specific time period.

A case that rings in my mind has to do with a 34-year-old woman with a successful law practice who had definite improvement in her problems following an extensive session with me a few years ago. She returned for a second session, which also went well. Following the removal of extraterrestrials, her Spirit Guide said that she will have a future life on another planet, so we decided to visit that life.

Her initial impression was that she and others on that planet looked somewhat human, were tall, around six feet, with thicker skin. She felt that the inhabitants of that planet were more evolved than we are on Earth, as she noticed that her bone joints were working better than normal. She answered many of my questions, namely that this was a peaceful planet with no war, no illness, and no obesity, and because of these things, these extraterrestrial beings have an extensive longevity, over two hundred Earth years. Also, all of their organs are strong and remain strong for long periods of time. Reproduction is similar to that which occurs on Earth; however, sexual intercourse occurs only when love is involved. Pregnancies last eight months instead of nine, as on Earth. Birth control is not used. Religion is non-existent, and almost everyone works.

The patient continued, "Our planet is natural and clean, with green oceans and yellow and orange landscape. There are very few animals, mostly domesticated ones who evolved with us. There are no buildings, and our houses are built into the ground. There are many millions of us on this planet, which is three times the size of Earth. When the inhabitants of this planet die, they are cremated, and the ashes are placed into the ground in a garden. There are no tombstones or graveyards. We do not have the technology to carry out space travel; however, the 'Gray Planet' does, by operating a spaceship shuttle which will take us and those from different planets to the Gray Planet or to other destinations."

I began to ask questions about the Gray Planet but could not believe what I was hearing. It was being described as if it was the 'playground of the universe.' My patient continued to speak from that lifetime, "If you want to be naughty, you go to the Gray Planet. It is smaller than Earth but much more advanced in technology of all sorts. They have everything, including large buildings, movies, drugs, gambling, cosmetic surgery, games, music, and food. They do not have war, but they do have crime, and their planet is nowhere as clean as ours. Our planet also has computers so we may communicate with the Gray Planet, thus we can easily go there to stay or for fun or go to other planets in the galaxy." Within six months of seeing this patient, I took another patient to a future life to a planet other than Earth, and once again heard about trips to the "Gray Planet, the playground of the universe."

LIFE ON A UTOPIAN PLANET

Another description of a future life involved a planet whose inhabitants were very humanoid-looking but with stronger features and were exceptionally tall, up to seven feet. Their genitalia and the process of reproduction were very similar to that of humans, and the inhabitants would intuitively know who they would reproduce with and raise a family with. These inhabitants also intuitively knew when their life was ending. At that time their soul entered another dimension, whereupon they could now incarnate to other planets. This planet is a three dimensional physical place, but the inhabitants are very spiritual and are able to do what a soul can do in the afterlife, namely think of being someplace and find themselves there. Communication is telepathic, worshipping God is primary, and love is the only emotion, which in my mind would explain why they have no war and live close to 500 Earth years. The population of this planet lives in peace with a global government and never experiences crime. This planet is not as large as Earth but has wonderful weather due to its having two suns and a large ocean. This utopian planet is one of many planets that are peaceful and without stress; however, I also hear words such as, "boring, not exciting, and lacking humor."

LIFE ON EARTH NOW AND IN THE FUTURE

Living on Earth currently offers a full range of emotions; therefore, people on Earth can be entertained and enjoy many parts of life, especially love, but in doing so we are open to the full gamut of problems that we face on Earth, namely war, disease, violence, crime, starvation, and every negative thought possible. As I have said before, life on Earth is not easy. One has to strive in many ways in order to live a joyful, happy life on Earth. In my mind this means encompassing spirituality and showing it, by loving and being kind to others. Living life on Earth in this way will help good overcome evil and hopefully unite humanity on battlefield Earth and truly bring peace to our planet in the future. This Earthly peace will supersede the peace that other planets have found because mankind will still have access to all its emotions, be able to have a world government, have enough spirituality to overcome entity attachment, and at the same time, maintain excitement, humor, entertainment, and yes, anything that's wholesome, positive, and contributes to one's joy and happiness in a good way.

FUTURE LIFE ON EARTH IN 2060

This particular patient, whose home was in Ontario, Canada, was instructed to go to a future life on Earth. He immediately saw himself in an extremely happy life in 2060, living in Australia. He was married and had four children. His chosen profession was that of being a successful architect.

I asked him to describe what life was like in the year 2060. He began slowly and then continued on ad infinitum. A lot of what I was hearing was what I have heard many times when patients experience a future life on Earth, especially during the years 2040 to 2060. Once again I was hearing that cars fly high in the year 2060, whereas twenty years earlier they were just able to hover; and at that time a cure for cancer was found. He said, "People would intuitively understand what's good and what's bad, and as a result, the entire planet enjoyed a great degree of happiness. Starvation did not exist, since food was grown on other planets and brought to Earth.

"Earth travel was carried out by individuals floating in a bubble that was small or as big as a house. One could travel from the east coast to the west coast of the United States in less than an hour. Ships still sailed the oceans, primarily for delivering cargo and for pleasure. There was no need for armies, just a police force in each country. The economy of the world remained good, and gold was no longer the standard, just paper.

"In regard to what people experienced in their personal lives in the year 2060, many of them lived in rather large town houses made of a special, durable glass. Food remained unchanged; it was just cooked longer, and therefore it was safer. Some drugs were legalized, but for the most part people decided not to use drugs. There were very few religions and very little interest in prostitutes and strip clubs. As people became more enlightened, the power of good won the battle against the power of evil, and the will of the people superseded the will of attached entities, whose number was dwindling, especially those of the dark forces. Thus, with fewer dark force attachments, there was much less evil in the world."

Chapter 11

PRESENT LIFE INFLUENCE

PRESENT DAY EMOTIONAL MEMORIES ALSO TAKE THEIR TOLL

Spirit Guides are unbelievably helpful when they show patients the reason that they are experiencing emotional suffering. They accomplish this by taking the patient back in time to the memory of a past event which was brought to the surface of the patient's subconscious mind by something that occurred in his present life. Most often it's a memory of an event from a past lifetime that took place with lots of emotion; however, the original event can also have occurred in the person's present lifetime. Occasionally there are several present-life occurrences that contribute to the problems that these types of patients are experiencing, all of which have caused the emotional problem to surface and be intensified. Taking the patient back to these interim occurrences won't cure the problem, but asking the Spirit Guide to take the patient back to the original cause, will. I have seen many patients whose emotional problem originated from an event that occurred in their present life. Sometimes these emotional problems may lead to physical problems, which can also improve when the original cause is brought up by the subconscious mind. Once the conscious mind sees the cause for what it truly is and understands clearly why it has affected him, it makes a judgment and is able to release the effect.

THE POWER OF PARENTS

Emotional past life memories can cause significant problems for a patient following a re-stimulation of this memory by someone or something in the patient's present life. By the same token, re-stimulation of an emotional memory from one's present life can also cause a person to suffer and sometimes to a greater degree. This type of situation often involves actions or comments from one's parents. As an obstetrician I have witnessed comments ranging from extremely negative to absolutely furious from fathers regarding their newborn baby because it was not the sex they had hoped for. These fathers did not seem to realize that such statements are being picked up and stored in the baby's subconscious mind. I have the same feelings about this type of parent as I had about abusive husbands and boyfriends when I practiced obstetrics and gynecology.

Some of the stories that I have heard from patients would make one's hair stand on end. To be told as a child by unthinking parents, "You're stupid!" or "You'll never amount to anything," or "You will never be happy," is a major devastation to a child in many ways, affecting his ego, his self-esteem, his confidence, his sense of fairness, his understanding of love and lack of it, and almost every aspect of his personality.

Children enjoy the sweetness of life until they hear such statements from a parent. Why does the child's blissful feeling vanish? How important, and how influential can words from one's parent be? From the perspective of one who has had twenty-three years of experience dealing with the subconscious mind under hypnosis, I would say unbelievably important and exceptionally influential. A child's ego can wave off negative comments from other children and even adults, but not from a person who loves you and cares for you.

Following such statements, a parent becomes one who is supposed to love you but is not apparently showing it. When a parent suspends rational judgment and makes such statements, his child can be so devastated that recovery may never happen and his or her life may never be the same again. This scenario can also occur when one parent decides to just pick up and leave the family or become abusive, verbally, physically, or sexually. The resulting emotional pain increases massively if both parents are contributing to such abuse.

As a result the child loses his self-esteem and self-confidence, feels he is never going to be good enough, and no one really cares how he feels. These feelings and deficits remain with him into adulthood and often lead to anxiety, depression, lack of motivation and energy, addictions, and a host of physical and emotional maladies. In addition to all this, the child within the adult person holds on to its pain.

Some of these adult patients who have undergone such abuse as a child also had similar and exceptionally deplorable past life memories surface, due to this present life abuse which served as a trigger to recall a very negative emotional past life memory which was buried in the subconscious mind. The degree of suffering that these individuals experience is hard to imagine. The original cause of the patient's problem is often found to be the subconscious recall of disturbing past life memories; however, when the patient is a child, and there is ongoing trauma from abusive parents, this situation should be considered a secondary cause and dealt with as well.

When adult patients with such problems undergo Comprehensive Hypnoregression Therapy, they become enlightened and begin to understand reincarnation and that they are eternal beings who have chosen this incarnation on Earth so as to learn lessons which will accelerate the process of perfecting their soul so they may eventually once again be One with the Creator. These patients will also come to understand that they chose this lifetime and everything that goes with it, including their parents, all for the purpose of learning certain lessons in this lifetime. I often remind the patient that forgiveness might just be one of those lessons. The patient's Spirit Guide is very helpful during the regression session and will usually allow the patient to look over the blueprint that he made for himself for this lifetime. It contains the lessons he needs to learn and helps the patient to gain insight.

Once all foreign energy has been evaluated, removed, and found not to be related to the patient's problem, the Spirit Guide is asked to take the patient back to the original cause of his problem and any lifetimes that have contributed to the patient's issues. Following an objective review of such an abusive event, the patient is now made to understand how important forgiveness is, especially the fact that it is done for the benefit of the patient, not the abuser. It is comparable to removing chains of unforgivingness which have continued to weigh the patient down and often lead to illness. The patient is then encouraged to truly forgive his parent or parents and make it come from the depths of his heart, and at the same time forgive himself for harboring all those negative thoughts about himself for many years. The patient must now understand that he is good enough and extremely worthy.

I remember a similar case involving dual hypnosis when my assistant's Spirit Guide said in regard to the patient, "He needs to love himself and others unconditionally. He needs to empower himself, not accept rejection, and be free to be himself. It's time to let go of the anger toward himself and others. What he thinks and feels does matter. He is not invisible. He will no longer be negative or say the words 'afraid of' or 'fear.' He needs to say, 'I can do better' and 'I am doing better.' He needs to feel the Light and love of God within him and have a knowing that he has the power to stand up to whatever he thought he feared and never be afraid to speak what he feels."

Following such sessions, patients will often feel like they are a brand new, very positive, and extremely happy person who is now enjoying life. I have even had such patients tell me that they sang and laughed all the way home following the session.

As a person grows up and continues contact with an abusive parent, he is allowing himself to bring up those negative memories over and over from his present day childhood and causing himself to continue living an extremely unhappy life. Patients who have separated from–or kept contact to a minimum–with such a parent or parents, and have forgiven them, have given themselves the greatest chance of happiness in this lifetime and hopefully are able to become good parents and raise their family in a loving manner. Such a path is easier to follow if patients are spiritually enlightened and won't permit negative people, even their own parents, to drain their positive energy. My regression therapy practice has uncovered an unbelievable number of horrible childhoods that patients have barely survived. It makes one thankful that he was fortunate enough to have a good childhood and grow up in a household with two loving parents.

RESURFACING OF CHILDHOOD FEARS FROM ONE'S PRESENT LIFE

The present economic downturn that is being experienced in America in the beginning of the 21st century, with its inevitable loss of peoples' savings, loss of jobs, and loss of homes, has served as a powerful, emotionally-negative stimulus to the subconscious minds of many individuals. This powerful stimulus has ignited many emotional and fearful childhood memories and has caused them to surface from the very depths of the subconscious mind. This situation wreaks havoc with the person's mental state and causes great suffering in the form of chronic anxiety, depression, insomnia, panic attacks, extreme nervousness, and all sorts of physical ramifications, such as hypertension, chest pain, gastrointestinal disorders, migraine headaches... the list is endless. I have regressed many of these patients who, when asked to go back to the cause, have gone back to the initial emotional event that occurred in their present childhood. Thus elderly patients who have lost their retirement or savings from massive present-day declines in the stock market are subconsciously recalling the childhood memories of the trauma their parents went through when they lost everything in the crash of 1929.

The great majority of these highly emotional past events occurred in prior lifetimes; however, there were a great deal of cases that pointed to present life problems as the original cause. Several cases had to do with people being upside down in their mortgage and therefore facing foreclosure and the loss of their home. This type of stress digs its tentacles into one's family, making the breadwinner feel like a failure and a loser, and in the process produces a variety of physical and emotional problems, as I have previously mentioned. The cases that I recall involved anxiety, depression, abdominal discomfort, and insomnia and required massive amounts of medications dispensed by a variety of physicians. The medications were minimally effective. Several cases that involved foreclosures had very similar original causes that had to do with traumatic divorce situations that the patient's parents went through when the patient was very young. At that time, each of these patients found himself in an emotionally jolting position of having to choose who he was to live with following their parents' divorce. This extremely disturbing moment in time caused each of them to be inundated with the fear of losing one of his parents, someone he loved very much. Their present mortgage crisis and potential loss of their home could bring on the subconscious fear of losing a loved one again, namely, their spouse, through a devastating separation or divorce. While in the altered state of hypnosis, the conscious minds of these patients were easily able to understand why the frightening foreclosure scenario resurrected the painful childhood memory that took place earlier in their present lives. As usual, their Spirit Guides were exceptionally helpful and instructed the patients to love, trust, and have faith in their families through thick and thin. I continue to be gratified by the improvement that the patients report upon follow up.

Chapter 12

PATIENTS WHO HAVE HAD REINCARNATIONS AS FAMOUS PEOPLE

ONE OF MY MOST MEMORABLE CASES

Several years ago Gerald, a very kind and intuitive gentleman called me from Toronto, Canada, to see if I could help him recover from the devastating effects of a stroke. I told him that I would do whatever I could to help him, and he then told me he could come and stay with relatives in Las Vegas during the time that I would be working with him. When Gerald arrived for his appointment, I was utterly impressed with his intelligence. He presented with a variety of physical and emotional problems, many of which were related to the onset of his stroke. His history brought out the fact that he had been very successful in his business ventures. It seems that he had an uncanny talent that allowed him to recognize patterns and be able to foretell the success or failure of various businesses. He said that he also made good use of astrology to help with these predictions.

The patient slipped easily into deep hypnosis and was hypnotically taken up to his Higher Self. Calls for his Spirit Guide were unsuccessful. Working with his Higher Self, I decided to take the patient back to a lifetime that would help explain his ability to predict future events. Immediately following this instruction, Gerald found himself in a dark room with many shelves containing metaphysical books and a gas lamp. In this 20th-century lifetime he was a man in his early thirties wearing slacks and a long-sleeved shirt. When I tried to advance the patient in time he immediately said that he had left this body and was in spirit form. I then asked him to return to that body, but instead he found himself in a different body at a much earlier time in a room with many books, but now the books had wooden covers. He described himself as a man in his early sixties who was looking out a window opening in a stone wall. He could see the ocean and hills and a castle through this window opening. He was wearing what seemed like a robe. As he looked around the room he noticed geometrical and planetary devices and various potions, as well as historical diaries of planetary movement and occurrences, some being in Arabic. Many of these big books had straw ties in their binding. He had the feeling that he was the one who had recorded and stored these records of events and occurrences. I asked what his name was; his response was, "Merlin."

 co℃ x 2ഗ

When people hear the name Merlin, they immediately associate him with Camelot, King Arthur, knights of the round table, and Lancelot, all of which they have been led to believe is mythology. Several authors have delved deeply into the possibility that Arthur did exist, Camelot was a real place, and individuals such as Merlin and Lancelot were also very real. Some of these authors claim to use archeological and documentary evidence to prove their case. One of these well-researched books was written by Rodney Castleden. It was entitled King Arthur: The Truth Behind the Legend.

co℃ x 2ഗ

Advancing the patient to when he was having a meal, he found himself in a great hall where there were many men with fancy uniforms wearing swords and armor. He immediately realized that he is a counsel and advisor for King Arthur, whom he recognized out in a courtyard by a garden. Arthur was dressed in black and was having a conversation with Sir Lancelot and a woman with red hair. They were discussing Merlin's prediction of an impending Viking invasion.

Advancing the patient to the next significant moment, Merlin saw himself on a hill with King Arthur and his army, looking for Viking ships as Merlin had predicted. By the middle of the day, three Viking ships had arrived, and Viking warriors were making their way to shore and heading for the villages upon landing. Arthur ordered his army to attack the Vikings, and as the battle raged on, Arthur, Lancelot, and Merlin watched from the hill. Arthur's forces finally overcame the Vikings and their leader, Dragar. Following the battle Arthur's army returned to his castle and surrounding village which was almost two days' inland by horseback.

After a victory celebration in the great hall, Merlin once again spent time in his special room carefully calculating planetary and geographical alignment so he may have more answers for Arthur about the future, and especially future conflicts. Arthur was very concerned that civil unrest will be coming to his kingdom. Merlin said, "Yes, there will be civil unrest, and it will be because of a famine which will soon be upon us."

In the coming year the early stages of a food shortage began to take place, mostly due to food taken by the Vikings during a multitude of small raids upon the villagers. A famine descended upon the villagers as the summer drought dragged on. This famine did not affect Arthur's castle or the surrounding villages; however, there were riots occurring in other villages. Arthur pressed Merlin for more answers. Merlin's response was that this famine will have to run its course, which may take a year and a half. Merlin also felt that Arthur will have to equitably distribute food to stop the unrest. Arthur agreed, but many of the knights did not. Merlin said that Arthur had no choice but to defeat the other knights. These rebellious knights joined together to fight Arthur and Lancelot. As a large battle ensued, Arthur decided to pull back and split his army in half. He then sent the first half of his army on a specific mission to invade the homeland of the knights and defeat them, castle by castle. The other half of Arthur's knights were to remain and fight the leaders who were now defeating them. During the height of this battle, the leaders of the rebellious knights broke off their offensive and returned home with their knights to defend their castles, thus allowing Arthur's army to be victorious. The other half of Arthur's forces took castle after castle and defeated these returning knights but allowed them to keep their castles, as long as they agreed to distribute food to the other villages. With this issue resolved, peace was restored for many years. Eventually Sir Lancelot left, and King Arthur died.

Advancing Merlin to the day of his death, his spirit left his body and remained in the lower astral plane. The Light did not appear to Merlin, and the thought that permeated his soul was that he really didn't want to leave the castle and all his possessions that helped him determine the future. He felt that he was different and stronger and didn't have to go to the Light. Merlin also remembered that when he was alive, he often heard a voice telling him that he didn't have to go to the Light if he didn't want to, and he could incarnate from the lower astral plane if he had the strength and knowledge. These strong thoughts came to him his whole life while meditating, but deep down Merlin knew that these thoughts were negative, probably coming from occult forces from the other side, and therefore were not true. Still, Merlin knew he was strong enough to find a way to live a life on Earth again.

Gerald spontaneously returned to the present time, and while still under deep hypnosis said his obsession with prophesying that originated in his life as Merlin is also the cause of his interest in Edgar Cayce. He then said, "I think I was also Edgar Cayce."

For those of you who are not familiar with Edgar Cayce, I would like to give you a little background on a man who became a very famous and extraordinary American with enviable personal integrity. In spite of never advancing beyond grammar school, he was extremely intelligent and enlightened and had psychic gifts which he unselfishly used to help others spiritually and medically. The most prominent, influential, and famous people of his day, including world leaders, would seek his advice. People made fortunes from his psychic talents, yet he lived simply, never seeking wealth or publicity.

Edgar Cayce was born in 1877 and died in 1945. For over forty years he was known as 'the sleeping prophet.' He would take himself into a deep altered state of consciousness and communicate with what he called "The Source." During these sessions he would have a stenographer present and an assistant who conducted the readings by transmitting information to him about individuals who had health problems or just wanted a "life reading." Given just a name and the location of the person with the problem, he would be able to come up with a diagnosis and a treatment, all of which came from The Source. His recommendations for treatment worked over 90% of the time, and he often said that if someone was ever hurt because of his treatment, he would stop doing this. His many thousands of treatments consisted of various concoctions using natural ingredients.

Edgar befriended the Blumenthal brothers, who were Wall Street stockbrokers. They engaged in readings with Edgar, resulting in guidance and insights which helped them to maintain their health and to become quite successful in their brokerage business. They were very grateful and eventually built the Cayce Hospital in Virginia Beach, Virginia, as The Source had recommended, so people could have their treatments administered exactly as told to Edgar by The Source. The first patient was admitted to the Hospital in February of 1929. During Edgar's readings for the Blumenthal brothers, The Source issued warnings of an impending upheaval in the stock market. The Blumenthal brothers did not heed the warnings and experienced heavy losses during the stock market crash that occurred on October 29, 1929. As a result, the Cayce Hospital closed shortly thereafter.

The Association for Research and Enlightenment (ARE) was formed at Virginia Beach, Virginia, in 1931. Their objective was to make all the data in Edgar Cayce's file of over 90,000 pages available to its membership and other groups in many cities. Many books, programs, lectures, and conferences have occurred under the auspices of the Association. I have the feeling that the ARE was the long-term goal of what Edgar Cayce referred to as The Source, who allowed the Blumenthal brothers to become wealthy and build the Cayce Hospital, which later was shut down. This same hospital building was eventually re-bought by Edgar Cayce supporters and in 1956 became the headquarters for ARE, which continues to be the main resource for thousands of study groups throughout the world.

Edgar Cayce felt that he was given a gift, that of helping people in a very unique way, and he felt compelled to help as many people as he could. As he got older, he felt that time was running out. In his prime, Edgar normally conducted two to three readings per day, but now that he was in his sixties, he was taking on five, six, or sometimes even seven cases a day. Edgar's compassionate desire to help people caused his overloaded schedule to take a toll on his health, and his family insisted that a reading be done on him. During that reading The Source told him that if he didn't slow down, he would die. Edgar remained selfless and continued to feel that people really needed his help, so he chose to continue with what he was doing, namely working compulsively and not resting, in spite of the warnings from The Source. Edgar developed pneumonia in February 1944 but continued to work relentlessly until he suffered a stroke in August of 1944, at which time his right side was paralyzed. A second stroke occurred shortly thereafter which resulted in paralysis of both sides of his body. One week before the second stroke he was able to do one final reading on himself. According to all that were present at that reading, the "Master of Masters" came through with advice for Edgar, which he also did not heed. Edgar Cayce's health steadily declined, and he died on January 3, 1945.

⁓

At the next session, I instructed Gerald to go back to a life as Edgar Cayce if such a life existed. The patient found himself to be a man in his fifties, walking on a beach in the northeastern United States. He made his way to his home, which was close to the beach, and described it as having brown shingles and vines. He was greeted by his wife and his teen-aged son as he entered his home. While he was in his house I asked him to look into a mirror and describe himself. He did so and said he's an older male who is balding. The patient then said that he thought he was a photographer and had spent a good bit of time alone in the dark with pictures. He also said that he could see colored auras in photographs that are brown and white, and these auras would lead to predictions. He also felt that he could intuitively tell things about people, whether they are good or evil, healthy or not.

At this point in the regression I again asked the patient to call forth his Spirit Guide and ask, "Will you help me?"

He then heard, "Use your magic."

I interrupted and said, "Why don't you draw on Merlin's talent?"

Following this, Gerald uttered the words, "Make it disappear," and almost immediately he found himself again on a beach, but this time it was a different beach, with very large and jagged rocks. It was cold and remote, and he was someone else, an adolescent male. Going along with the fact that the patient had jumped into a different past lifetime, I then advanced him to being in his home, which he described as a cabin with a big fireplace. His parents were there and referred to him as 'Boy.' I then asked him to tell his parents to please use his proper name. He then said they just laughed. The patient was twelve years old in this lifetime and had home schooling from his mother. His father was a blacksmith and could neither read nor write. When advanced to the age of 21, he saw himself in a learning institution in the British Isles learning the metaphysical arts. His name was Efram. When I asked for an overview of that life, he told me that the training was rather rigid and the students were not allowed to read for themselves, rather they were only allowed to be read to, and thus he could only retain information from memory. If a student was not successful at this, he was not permitted to continue with the program. Eventually he graduated and became a predictor, one of three priests who controlled the government of England. He died in his late fifties. Following his death he again did not perceive the Light and remained in the lower astral plane.

Gerald's Higher Self revealed the fact that he had the help of three mentors, all of whom were recognized authorities in the business world. These three mentors were deceased and somehow, as spirits, reinforced the patient's ideas and predictions; however, they were not attached.

I decided to once again call for a Spirit Guide. The patient's Higher Self said, "There is no Spirit Guide, but Nathan, one of the mentors, is here."

I then asked if there was anyone attached to the patient. The patient's mentor, Nathan, answered, "Gregory is coming through."

I then began to interrogate Gregory, who I suspected to be an Earthbound spirit. I asked, "How long have you been with him?"

He answered, "Fourteen years; I was sent by Nathan."

I pressed him further. "What is your purpose in being here?"

Gregory replied, "Time and space. I need him to understand this. We had a life together as acquaintances and had overlapping skills. Mine was time and space; his was Galileo type stuff."

I then asked what my patient's name was in that life. Gregory answered, "Edgar Cayce," and then said that my patient in his present life and in his life as Edgar Cayce often went to the Akashic Records to find knowledge. He would just call for the knowledge, and it appeared. (The Akashic Records are thought to be an etheric compilation of all the knowledge of all human existence that has ever occurred in time and space.)

Gregory had died of a heart attack and did not go to the Light; instead, he attached to my patient from the lower astral plane some fourteen years ago. I then asked Gregory how he has affected the patient. His answer was that his weak heart was imprinted upon the patient's body. Gregory then said, "I have to pass on the secret of the strings, and I am not leaving until I do this."

I replied, "Can you do this now?"

Gregory answered quickly. "He needs to hold on to the twos and sixes."

The patient became agitated, so I asked, "What's happening?"

This time Gerald's mentor Nathan spoke. "Gregory has gone to the Light." I again called for a Spirit Guide, but to no avail. Nathan spoke again, saying that he did not see any Spirit Guide appearing and that my patient did not need one and won't get one because he is attached to the Earth, to the lower astral plane, from which he cannot incarnate. Nathan continued, "He is grounded there; however, he can move on directly after death. He does not do this by incarnating, rather he is a Walk-in at birth. There are others like this. Most of them have innate special talents. They are driven; they are too busy to go to the Light. They may make agreements with souls about to be born in a new body, and thus they also can become First Soul in an infant. Others may join later as Walk-throughs, two or three or more. These are souls joining for a temporary period of time, and they can only join if they have an equal profile. A weak soul cannot walk through a strong soul. If it did, it would be sent back to the Light and have a difficult time incarnating. It would become a wanderer and may not find its way back. A weak soul means less accomplishment. It has to do with the development of the soul mind, which is like a snowball effect. Strong souls are the gross minority."

What I was hearing was literally blowing my mind. Nathan, a very advanced mentor, was clearly showing me very much needed and very much appreciated validation. Hearing what mentor Nathan had to say was causing my heart to beat faster. This was the second time that I was hearing the term "Walk-through." The first time was as a gift from a Spirit Guide. Occasionally a Spirit Guide will say to me, "I have a gift for you," and make me aware of an important piece of the spiritual puzzle that will help me to better understand the spiritual world and thus enable me to do more for my patients. Some time ago I was given a gift of spectacular information wherein a Spirit Guide made me aware of the Walk-through phenomenon. This particular gift was explained to me in great detail by the Spirit Guide who indicated that a soul (Soul A) may need to learn a specific lesson from a certain perspective and therefore not incarnate immediately, but instead look over the Akashic records. By doing so, this soul (Soul A) may then decide to access a portion of another soul's experience (Soul B) for the period of time needed to learn its lessons. Thus, Soul A makes an agreement with Soul B and obtains permission to occupy the same body that Soul B occupies, for a temporary period of time. The Spirit Guide insisted that this should be looked upon as a visitation, to pick up on all the facets of Soul B's lifetime so Soul A can fulfill his need to learn a specific lesson from Soul B's perspective.

At that time I asked if Soul B was a high-profile soul, or in other words, a famous person. The Spirit Guide answered quickly, saying, "Yes, there is no need to visit a life which is spiritually stagnant and without challenge. The goal of enlightenment, of experience, of actualization, is to be where the action is. It's where the energy is, it's where the focus is, it's where the soul needs to be."

The Spirit Guide compared the Walk-through phenomenon to the Walk-in phenomenon, wherein a soul with a body makes an agreement to switch places permanently with a soul without a body. Both phenomena require a mutual permission agreement between souls. The motive of a Walk-in is usually to help humankind;

however, the Walk-through is just that, it's a temporary period of Earth-time for one soul to "visit" with another soul in the same body for the purpose of learning a particular lesson through that original soul's perspective, and then leave.

I am now being told by Gerald's mentor Nathan that the Walk-through phenomenon always involves a soul who is famous in his own right (Soul A), experiencing, walking through, or sharing the body of another famous person (Soul B) while that famous person's soul remains in place. Thus the visiting high profile Soul A can absorb the energy and the experience of the other high profile original Soul B.

This information enabled me to finally fill in the blanks for a problem that I had no answers for, namely being able to historically validate past lifetimes of people who saw themselves as a famous person in history. I can now do this with the understanding that the validation may end at a certain point in that life because that particular person was a Walk-through soul. I have had a few of these cases, including a patient who was Jim Thorpe, an Olympic star. I was able to validate a portion of this famous person's lifetime in that case, but when I reached a certain point in that lifetime, the validation ceased. I now know why; it was because my patient was a Walk-through and had left to begin his incarnation. Also, I have been told by the Spirit Guides of famous people that these high-profile individuals often had many souls in their body. I encountered one such case, that of a patient who was Joan of Arc in a past life. The patient's Spirit Guide said that she had many souls within her as she was being burned at the stake. My wife's comments on my work are often quite interesting. Her comment here was that having many advanced souls in a high-profile or famous person would provide additional perspectives and strength to the Original Soul, enabling him to perform beyond expectation, thus elevating his fame and assuring a permanent place in history.

I have had a considerable number of patients who have had reincarnations as famous people in history. These famous people, mentioned in my first book, include Joan of Arc, Goliath, William

James, Jim Thorpe, and several apostles. In this book I am add-
ing to the list Merlin, Edgar Cayce, Black Elk, St. Joseph, Doc
Holliday, and Marilyn Monroe.

This Walk-through phenomenon explains how several people
can claim to be the reincarnation of the same famous, or high-profile, historical person. This phenomenon can also apply to my present
case, since other people have asserted that they may be the reincarnation of Edgar Cayce. Some of their proof lies in the similarity of
personality, accomplishments, intelligence, gifts, and facial features.
If one considers the possibility that the Walk-through phenomenon
may truly be the way it is described by Spirit Guides and mentors
in the spiritual dimension, then several people may indeed have
experienced life as Edgar Cayce by joining him as a Walk-through.
However, one of the individuals may have been the original Edgar
Cayce who came into his life as a Walk-in, or more likely as a first
soul Walk-in at birth, and the others were Walk-throughs.

The mentor Nathan in the present case involving Edgar Cayce
said, "A weak soul cannot walk through a strong soul," and then
defined a strong soul as one with great accomplishments, or in other
words, a high profile or famous person. Once again we are being given
information that will help us understand the complexities of the spirit
world. Nathan was, in effect, telling us that a Walk-through phenomenon cannot occur if the entering soul has not had many accomplishments which have to do with the development of the soul mind. I
interpret this to mean a soul which has raised its vibration by accomplishing the learning of many lessons throughout its incarnations,
making it a "strong soul." It is good to see consistency in terminology
with regard to the Walk-through phenomenon coming from different
patients' Spirit Guides and mentors. In my mind, this is validation.

❧

At my patient's last session, I once more instructed him to go back to
a life as Edgar Cayce, if it indeed existed, and enter into that lifetime

at a significant moment. The patient immediately found himself on a couch. He was a man in his sixties, alone, not awake, and not asleep. He was in a hypnotic trance state. The mentor Nathan began to describe what was happening. "Edgar Cayce is in a focused state, focusing on the Akashic records in an attempt to find answers to what caused the destruction of Atlantis."

While in trance, Edgar Cayce began to speak. "I see many things during this pursuit, including earthquakes with plates separating; volcanoes erupting; step-stage pyramids (not smooth sided) being used for protection from gravitational pull; crystals within the pyramids being used for longevity; and crystal skulls being used by mystics for consciousness transference. I am beginning to absorb knowledge, much like the original settlers from space did, in the form of spirits who took over bodies at will. Man was too primitive to disagree. As man developed, spirits locked in, bodies eventually died, and spirits took another body. Man soon developed his own spirit. When one dies, his weak soul may or may not strengthen in the afterlife. This has been happening even in present day. Modern man is mostly aboriginal. There are too many unspecial souls. They are like lemmings (followers), little rodents who blindly follow their leaders off of a cliff or into water, where they die.

"In Lemuria spirits went to bodies but could go back and forth from the spirit form. Spirits liked the bodies so much that they became trapped in those bodies. Lemuria was eventually disbanded, and people went to other continents.

"The Earth is still growing and shifting. There is no line-up problem. Atlantis was more of a volcanic problem. Cultures in ancient times were near volcanoes, so people could have a geothermal power source. They used it to generate a turbine effect. The people leaving took the knowledge with them, but not the technology. The original spirits have their own source of energy; others had volcanoes and rivers."

As I was listening intently and taking notes from this alleged Edgar Cayce in trance, I came up with an awesome idea. Why not prove my patient was Edgar Cayce, and what better way than to have him cure a medical problem while in trance? I had been suffering from a large bone spur on my ankle for over a year. It had grown to about three centimeters and was extremely painful when walking. Having been Chief of Surgery, I was aware that surgery was not a good option. The individuals that I saw undergo orthopedic or podiatric surgery for this problem weren't able to walk for a considerable amount of time following surgery, and when they did, their gait was sometimes altered. I thus decided to ask about a treatment for my enlarged, painful bone spur. The treatment that he came up with as Edgar Cayce consisted of using a combination of olive oil, the spice turmeric, and a few drops of DMSO (dimethyl sulfoxide), to get it quickly absorbed. I applied this several times a day for several months. My bone spur became smaller and smaller, and by the end of six months it was practically non-existent.

The case I have just presented adds credence to the method in which more advanced souls handle reincarnation. Following physical death, they do not go to the Light from where they can carry out traditional reincarnation, but rather they choose to remain in the lower astral plane. Advanced souls arrange a Walk-in agreement soon after death, or as soon as possible, with another living human being. These advanced souls do this so they may complete their unfinished business and be able to continue the good work they have been doing. If the person who agrees to the Walk-in arrangement is an older child or an adult, the advanced soul would know that his agenda would not be easily carried out due to the desires and personality already present in that body. I have been told that these advanced souls often prefer to enter a new body that is about to be born and thus become first soul in an infant. This enables them to have a greater opportunity to carry out their good work without interference. I would think that such Walk-in agreements could also be made within hours of a baby's birth with the same effect, namely, for the highly advanced Walk-in soul to fully imprint its personality and the priorities that it needs to pursue within this new body's consciousness.

Advanced souls may decide to delay their entrance into the physical world through a Walk-in agreement and instead temporarily attach as Earthbound spirits to a living person whom they feel will be easily influenced and inspired to carry out their agenda and unfinished business. When they decide to leave their hosts, they will then enter the physical world as a Walk-in, and if possible, a first-born Walk-in. My thoughts on this subject are that souls who are advanced in spiritual terms are often the same individuals who are famous in Earthly terms, by possessing talent and gifts that are way beyond normal human ability.

My patient Gerald, Merlin, and Edgar Cayce, all seemed to be surrounded with similarities that reek of synchronicity. All three were very gifted and were able to foretell the future. All three were involved with astrology (Edgar Cayce's comments regarding astrology occurred during trance states), and all were compulsive about getting done what needs to be done. Both Gerald and Edgar Cayce suffered strokes and eventually died at home in their sixties.

The case we have been discussing is quite unusual in that the patient, when taken back to the source of his prophesying, went back to his life as Merlin. Following his regression to that life, the patient said he was utterly fascinated with Edgar Cayce and his gift of precognition. He then said, "I think I was also Edgar Cayce." We then took him back to that lifetime. Edgar Cayce validated his presence by coming through with a successful treatment for a painful bone spur that I had, by recommending a treatment consisting of a concoction of natural ingredients that worked. This was a first for me, to have a patient return to two lifetimes as famous people.

I am sure Edgar Cayce's soul was as compulsive in the lower astral plane as it was when he was in a physical human body. If this was true, and he needed to get back into a physical body soon so he could continue to help people, it would stand to reason that he would rather choose the preferable route, that of a Walk-in, as First Soul in an infant. This theory is a possibility, but it is a strong possibility, since Edgar Cayce died on January 3, 1945, the same day my patient, Gerald, was born, an ideal time for a newborn Walk-in.

THE NATIVE AMERICAN KNIGHT

This middle-aged, well-educated male patient from Philadelphia came to me to resolve a question in his mind. He had always had a tremendous interest in anything Native American. His mother told him that as soon as he could walk and talk, he wanted to be an Indian. As an adult, he has been carrying out "flint knapping" and archery and only hunts game with a bow and arrow and does so successfully. A question in his mind began to surface after he read *Bury My Heart at Wounded Knee* and wept uncontrollably. These highly emotional reactions remained disturbingly consistent as he continued to read other books about the Lakota Sioux, Ishi, Apache, and the Navajo Indians. However, when he read *Black Elk Speaks*, he began to identify with Black Elk, the Lakota Sioux warrior who fought at the battles of Little Big Horn and Wounded Knee. Thus the question that continued to haunt his consciousness was, had he been Black Elk in that lifetime?

Following induction into deep hypnosis, two attempts at locating his Spirit Guide failed, and the patient kept saying, "My right brain can't function; it's bound up."

Finally I was successful at getting the Spirit Guide on board. When I asked about the presence of foreign energy, the Spirit Guide replied, "There is a net around him, and it's dark."

I then conducted an exorcism and had the net encapsulated in Light and then removed by St. Michael the Archangel. When I asked the Spirit Guide about more foreign energy being present, I was told, "I can't tell." This wasn't good enough. I need valid and unequivocal confirmation of what's happening during entity releasement, so I then invoked the additional help of Abel, my volunteer Spirit Guide who often shows up when I call him. Abel came forth

WHAT'S MISSING IN MEDICINE

and immediately spotted a demonic Reptilian extraterrestrial. Once again I conducted an exorcism and the Reptilian was encapsulated with Light and taken to the Light by St. Michael the Archangel. No implants were present. Right after that transpired, the patient yelled out, "My right brain is free!"

I then asked Abel, my volunteer Spirit Guide, to take the patient back to a life as Black Elk, if such a life existed. The patient uttered softly, "I *was* Black Elk," and with tears flowing he continued, "I am at Wounded Knee, and there are people dead everywhere." During that regression he also confirmed that his deceased brother, Albert, was Crazy Horse, the Sioux chief in that lifetime. History shows that Black Elk accompanied his good friend, Crazy Horse, on a trip to Fort Robinson in Nebraska to negotiate peace. Crazy Horse was bayoneted and murdered at the age of 30 when he went to meet the commanding officer. Spirit Guide Abel then opened up the blueprint that Black Elk made for himself when he incarnated into this lifetime. The lesson that he needed to learn was, "No matter how hard things are, you can help others." This lesson was accomplished. Black Elk eventually settled in South Dakota and died August 18, 1950. My patient was born November 18, 1950.

UNCONDITIONAL LOVE FOR JESUS

The case that I am about to present involved an extremely gifted young woman from New York City by the name of Jessica. Her gifts included occasionally seeing auras around people, specific kinds of precognition, and the ability to feel various forms of energy. As soon as Jessica was taken into deep hypnosis, her Spirit Guide, Acetar, made his entrance and informed me that he had been with her for over three hundred years. When I asked about foreign energy being present, his answer was no. He also indicated that he has had many lifetimes with her. Following this statement I asked if he could take us back to one of those lifetimes that was rather significant. Almost immediately Jessica found herself in an ancient lifetime as an old man with a cane, wearing a maroon robe. As she assumed that person's mind, body, and memories in that life, she softly exclaimed, "I'm St. Joseph!"

Advancing St. Joseph to the next significant moment, he found himself leading many people to Jerusalem so they may see and hear Christ. Upon arriving in Jerusalem, St. Joseph saw Jesus and felt unconditional love as his tears of happiness flowed freely. Jessica openly cried as she described the radiant white and pink Light around Jesus. St. Joseph then said, "Jesus brought hope and the Word of God to the people. I have accomplished what I needed to do; I brought many people to see Him." At that moment another Spirit Guide by the name of Sonitor arrived and said he had been with Jessica for all eternity. Sonitor informed us that St. Joseph died in a cave at the age of 86 and had accomplished his lesson, that of unconditional love.

GUNFIGHT AT THE O.K. CORRAL

This very colorful gentleman came to me from North Dakota with an extensive list of physical and emotional ailments as well as addictions, whereby he considered himself a multiple-substance abuser. His Spirit Guide was readily available under deep hypnosis and confirmed the release of many dark force entities along with a half-dozen Earthbound spirits who contributed heavily to his alcohol and drug addictions.

This patient felt very strongly that he was Doc Holiday in a past lifetime and that a particular woman in his present life was Katherine "Kate" Hornsby, a prostitute who befriended Doc Holiday in that past lifetime in the mid-1800s. The patient's Spirit Guide confirmed this and helped me take the patient back to several events that occurred in Doc Holiday's life.

These incidents in the life of Doc Holiday included his early teenage years which found him to be very proficient with a long-barreled six gun and utterly remorseful following his mother's death.

His father was very loose with women and remarried within three months of her death.

Several years later Doc Holiday moved to Georgia and attended dental school. He practiced for a few years and then moved to Texas, where he spent a lot of time gambling. By this time he had become a flaming alcoholic and began to suffer from tuberculosis. He often felt weak and sick and bore a great deal of physical pain that worsened when he walked on the stones on the road or rode his horse. This pain even surfaced when he was walking over the squeaking irregularities on the wooden walkways that lay on each side of the dirt road in town.

He became involved in many altercations involving guns, especially with gamblers, and always came out on top. Because of this, Doc Holiday eventually became a wanted man but somehow managed to continue to practice his dental trade.

I was always excited about the shootout at the O.K. Corral in Tombstone, so I advanced the patient to that event, which found Doc Holiday talking to his good friend Wyatt Earp about the hostility of the local cowboys who were presently threatening them. Doc and Wyatt were joined by Wyatt's older brother, Virgil, a deputy U. S. Marshall, and Wyatt's younger brother, Morgan, as they walked slowly towards the O.K. Corral where five cowboys were waiting for them. Doc had been made a temporary deputy of Virgil's. When they arrived there was a plethora of silence as each man stared at the men opposing them. This abruptly ended when Doc decided to cock his shotgun. This sudden move set into motion a flurry of gunshots from both sides. When the smoke settled, Morgan was wounded, Virgil was hurt badly, Doc was grazed, and three of the cowboys lay dead.

SOME LIKE IT HOT

Renee was an attractive twenty-two-year-old woman from Ontario, Canada, who came to see me with the complaint that something was missing in her life. She felt that this missing link had to do with a future career, something she would be passionate about and something that would bring her extreme happiness. I was fortunate to locate a most helpful Spirit Guide with extensive experience. The Spirit Guide took the patient back to the cause of this feeling, and we entered the lifetime of the famous actress of the 1950s, Marilyn Monroe. The patient confirmed many aspects of that lifetime, including much of which has already been written about. When taken to her death experience, she insisted that she did not commit suicide and that a man in a dark hat and a long, dark coat broke into her room and forced her to take an overdose of sleeping pills. The Spirit Guide said that her lesson in that lifetime was to love herself unconditionally. This was not accomplished, and so remains as one of the lessons that she needs to learn in her present life. The patient felt that she always had a passion to entertain and that this was the missing link she was searching for.

⚜

My experience with patients who were famous in other lives and my knowledge of the walk-though phenomenon has led me to believe that famous people who have attained their prominence in various disciplines seem to have something in common besides having accomplished a great deal in their chosen field. They often feel that their death came too soon and that they had more to accomplish. This powerful energy that they have harnessed continues on within their consciousness as a fervent desire to complete unfinished business and often causes them to decline going to the Light following death, and thus remain in the lower astral plane. It seems that they would then seek out individuals who are alive and talented and either join them as an uninvited attachment for the purpose of inspiring them to hopefully accomplish and complete many of the things that they were unable to, or carry out a Walk-in arrangement with a soul who has a living body, preferably at birth.

Chapter 13

WALK-INS

As mentioned in the previous chapter, "Walk-in" is the term given to the phenomenon wherein a soul without a living body exchanges places with a soul who has its own living human body. Both souls carry out this exchange by mutual agreement. The term 'Walk-in' was coined by Ruth Montgomery, a very enlightened and renowned author, in her book *Strangers Among Us*, which was published in 1979 and delves deeply into the concept of Walk-ins. Ruth Montgomery's information was channeled through Guides:

"Her Guides had described Walk-ins as souls who have earned the right, through many lifetimes of spiritual growth, to return directly to the earth plane as adults, by taking over unwanted bodies if their intent is to help mankind. Sometimes the original occupant has become so dispirited that he or she wishes to bow out. In other cases, an accident or severe illness has damaged the body to such an extent that its inhabitant can no longer maintain the spark of life.

" 'These Walk-ins,' the Guides declared, 'are not yet perfected souls, but are high-minded beings intent on aiding their fellow humans, and tens of thousands of them are already here, not as towering leaders but as quiet helpers.' "[8]

---

8 Montgomery, Ruth, and Joanne Garland. *Ruth Montgomery: Herald of the New Age*, Fawcett Crest: NY, NY, 1986, p. 202-203.

" 'They are filled with a sense of purpose,' the Guides declared of Walk-ins, 'and an urgency to get on with the task of helping mankind and saving planet earth in these coming decades. They feel that time is short, and their frustration with their inability, at times, to discover their mission is self-evident.' Continuing, the Guides stressed, most Walk-ins are not busily asserting themselves and giving advice, but rather are 'gently guiding others in the path of fellowship and self-help.' "[9]

I rarely encounter such cases, but when I do, I find them most fascinating. Under deep hypnosis the patient's Spirit Guide, and sometimes his Higher Self, will relay the fact that he, the patient, was not born into this world but rather came in as a Walk-in. The patient can be taken back to the moment of the exchange so he can better understand his reason for being in this lifetime as that person. If necessary, he can also be regressed to when this agreement was made. The new soul will retain the memories of the original resident soul, but relationships with loved ones and other people will most likely be modified. The patient's Spirit Guide can be extremely helpful in these situations.

Some people feel that the incoming soul is obligated to pursue the goals that the original resident soul had. Others feel that the incoming soul is a very special soul that enters a human body for a very specific purpose, namely, to help people. In my experience I have found that the incoming soul is from someone who died on Earth or another planet or is from another dimension. I have also found that once the Walk-in soul has entered a body, that body is still vulnerable to entity infestation and is still weighed down by the entities that were attached before the soul exchange.

The previous chapter discussed in detail how the souls of famous or high-profile humans are often so befuddled with excessive unfinished business at death that they choose to not go to the Light and instead remain in the lower astral plane. Here they can eventually

---

9 Ibid. p. 211.

locate and attach to an individual with much potential, and hopefully have this person complete their unfinished business. If these high-profile souls, who are very enlightened and advanced in their accomplishments, are not successful in this pursuit, they may decide to reenter a life again as a Walk-in, preferably at birth, as a first soul. Their high-profile status will often act as a magnet and draw Walk-through souls who will then join with this high-profile soul in the same body for a temporary period of time for the purpose of learning lessons from his perspective.

NOT REALLY ABANDONED

Early in my career, and well before I began working with Spirit Guides and releasing attached entities, I encountered a case that involved a Walk-in. At that time I was only using hypnotic past life regression to help people rid themselves of their problems. This particular case was my first experience with a Walk-in situation. I had heard of such cases but had never run across one. At that time I would work with and communicate with the patient's Higher Self.

Diane was an attractive, intelligent, and spiritual woman in her early forties who came to me from El Paso, Texas, eager to rid herself of a depression problem. She turned out to be a good subject, and when instructed to go back to the cause of her depression, her facial expression took on a serious tone as tears formed in her eyes. Words slowly came out of her quivering mouth as she said, "I was abandoned on Earth."

At this moment I was very confused, and I asked many questions. It seems that she came from Lemuria, a realm with a higher vibration. The purpose of her coming to Earth was to be of assistance to Earthlings and help them with their problems. Her entryway into this physical world did not involve a birth process, rather her soul, which was body-less, made an agreement to change places with another soul who was in the body of a seventeen-year-old girl who wanted to leave Earth. This mutual soul agreement to change places was made in the spiritual dimension. I asked if she had any contact with or communication from Lemuria. The patient said no, but she felt the presence of elevated Master Spirits from other realms who seemed to be keeping an eye on her.

Diane confessed that she had forgotten who she was when she became this seventeen-year-old girl, and as such retained the memory of this girl's experiences. A prominent subconscious feeling that has remained with her since the Walk-in took place was the feeling that she had been abandoned. Diane's conscious mind was fully awake during the altered state of consciousness that occurs with hypnosis and was now able to understand that she was not abandoned and that she voluntarily entered this Earth life as a Walk-in with the charitable intent to aid fellow humans on Earth. Her conscious mind can also understand that her depression was occurring because of a subconscious feeling of abandonment which she was not consciously aware of. Now that she realizes who she is and understands the noble mission that she is on and the fact that she was never abandoned, her conscious mind can now make a judgment that there is no further reason for her to be depressed.

A big smile was evident upon waking from the session as Diane expressed that she was unbelievably surprised at what came forth from her subconscious mind. She also mentioned that her life took on a more spiritual tone at age 17. Since that time she has discovered that she has certain gifts that allow her to see and communicate with spirit entities and has helped them go to the Light. She also found that she can help people when she is engaged in an out-of-body experience. Diane did very well following this session, and I understand that as of two and a half years later, her depression has not returned.

THE MESSENGER

This fascinating case centers on Robert, a young man whose main concern was that his body has on occasion moved in unusual ways over the past six months. These bizarre movements started when the patient first began to utilize meditation to enhance his spirituality.

The patient's history brought to light many interesting facts, namely that he has always had a fascination with knighthood, that he has an innate knowledge of his being different from others, and that he has an inherent need to help people. In addition, my interview of this patient revealed the fact that he was very spiritually enlightened and that he felt his unusual body movements were somehow an expression of energy within him. He had a regression performed on him utilizing the computer program Skype several years ago which uncovered many lifetimes, including one as a knight. He also saw himself traveling in space with a distinct mission, that of helping people.

The patient's hypnotic induction was punctuated by varying degrees of rather extreme gyrating and undulating body movements, along with piercing sounds from his voice. As I witnessed this very strange reaction to induction, I remembered that the patient's unusual body movements began when the patient was meditating. My thoughts then went to the fact that brainwaves slow down when one goes from beta wave waking state to alpha wave meditation state. Now we are taking the patient into a hypnotic theta state, where the brainwaves run even slower. The patient's movements appeared to become more bizarre as I took him deeper but leveled off when I pressed on his forehead and relaxed him more.

Following hypnotic ascension into his Higher Self, I was able to communicate with his Spirit Guide who informed me that the patient did not have any foreign energy present and was not fragmented. When I asked the Spirit Guide about the patient's unusual movements, I was told that it is a manifestation of accumulated energy. The Spirit Guide then began to explain who Robert really is and what his mission is all about. The Guide said, "Robert is from another dimension and is a spiritual messenger from God, the Creator, the Source. Robert has entered this life to help people understand what they can do and what they can become. Robert is very sensitive and will feel people's pain as he teaches them; however, he will not be able to teach and help people until he learns to be human in each lifetime that he's in. He must first be among them, understand them, and be one of them for a certain period of time; only then will he be able to teach people, who will be able to teach others. Robert has incarnated into eighteen past lives for this purpose. He carried out these incarnations as a Walk-in, either as a child or as an adult. In his present life, his Walk-in occurred with a two-year-old boy.

"Robert does not die in any of these prior lifetimes, rather he just disappears and leaves this Earth in his thirty-third year. His present lifetime is his nineteenth and last reincarnation for this purpose. This is his last life on Earth. In this life he will go beyond thirty-three years on Earth. He will begin to lead in twenty years and will raise a family until then. Others like him will bring knowledge and help to certain people, who will become teachers and help others. These actions will shield people from dark force influence."

At this moment the patient, still under deep hypnosis, turned his head toward me and said, "When I was a little boy in another life you took me under your wing. You were a French knight, and I was drawn to you. I was a little boy in your village. You taught me to understand people and be fearless; you taught me to be a knight. Once again I am in your lifetime, and once again, I need to open up to what I will become in this lifetime. Once again you will teach me to become a knight and save people."

This is the third patient that shared my past life when I was a French knight. The first was Evelyn, a surgeon's secretary in Chardon, Ohio, who was my half-sister in that life. Her lifetime with me was validated by the Spirit Guide experiment that I carried out and talked about in my first book. The second patient that was in that life with me was a fellow knight who fought alongside me in many battles. Presently he has become a close friend. (I elaborated upon my past life as a French knight in Chapter Two, subtitled *Love Those Spirit Guides*.)

Chapter 14

DUAL HYPNOSIS

DUAL HYPNOSIS USING SOMEONE ACCOMPANYING THE PATIENT

CREATIVITY PAYS OFF

When I see a husband and wife in separate sessions and am only able to communicate with a Spirit Guide from one of them, I suggest that they return for a dual hypnosis session, providing they have no privacy issues. When they return for the dual session, I hypnotize them side by side, utilizing the one Spirit Guide for both of them and immediately check for the presence of foreign energy, always starting with dark forces and powerful dark forces. Thus in these cases I will conduct a dual hypnosis but start off with an exorcism to prevent the dark forces, and especially the powerful ones, from hiding, or keeping their frequencies from being identified by the Spirit Guide. I also feel that it is important to remove foreign energy from both spouses early on, since, as mentioned before, the powerful dark forces can hide and later be transferred from one spouse to the other through sexual intercourse.

If I am seeing a husband and wife for the first time, who arrive together, and each of them would like to have a session, I will often suggest that we conduct a dual hypnosis session to begin with, if there are no privacy issues. I do this so as to make the session more meaningful by doubling the likelihood of communicating with a valid Spirit Guide. Also I am often successful in taking both patients back to a life they shared, if such a life existed.

Having two Spirit Guides is great, but one is quite sufficient, and one is all I need to remove entities. As I said before, experience has taught me to always start entity removal by identifying and removing dark forces first. The reason for this is that dark forces, and especially powerful dark forces, seem to know when I am coming after them. Performing an exorcism for both patients simultaneously during dual hypnosis makes it much more difficult for dark forces to leave or hide. This type of session can be more complex, so the therapist must be well-organized and clear when speaking to the patients or their Spirit Guides. Such sessions work well and accomplish what's needed.

Patients will occasionally come in for a session and bring someone other than their spouse with them for moral support. The person who accompanies the patient will either be present for the session with the patient's consent, or he or she will remain in the waiting room. On occasion the patient may request that this person take part in a dual session with him. The dual session will then take place as long as everyone consents and there are no privacy issues.

If I am able to come up with at least one valid Spirit Guide, the session will usually go very smoothly. If, however, I am unable to access a valid Spirit Guide, or even my volunteer Spirit Guide, I immediately suspect dark forces and take the patient through powerful suggestions for the subconscious mind, instruct the patient in protective measures, and then bring them both out of hypnosis. I then let the patient know that I am 100% sure that we are dealing with many dark forces or powerful dark forces, and that I would like him to return for a dual hypnosis session with my assistant, who has an excellent Spirit Guide that consistently comes forth when called upon. I then let the patient know that I am fully confident that we will accomplish everything that's needed in this upcoming dual hypnosis session.

DUAL ABDUCTION

People will occasionally have conscious memory of an alien abduction. This particular case involves Edith and Peter, two people who saw each other for the first time during such an abduction. Three years later, this man and woman met each other for the first time, and each of them had an instant recognition of the other and a conscious memory of the circumstances that existed during their first meeting while being abducted by aliens. They have since developed a close relationship and have been comparing events and situations that have occurred in their lives that are rather paranormal. Because of the unusual circumstances under which this couple met, I decided early on to carry out a dual hypnosis on both of them simultaneously if they had no objection and no problem with privacy issues.

My interview with Edith revealed a phobia of darkness since childhood, hatred of owls and clowns, missing time, and a feeling of being pinned down and paralyzed in bed when awake, while the scent of sewer was very prominent. She described a recent sore on the popliteal area (back of the knee). After applying peroxide to it, this raw area bubbled, and she felt a hard, BB sized object which she removed and attempted to save; however, it quickly became jelly-like and dissolved (this is not the first time that I have heard about an extraterrestrial implant dissolving upon removal.) Edith woke up one week before her appointment with a cut on the inner curve of her ear. The laceration was still open when she showed me the area. She has witnessed several paranormal events in her home, including seeing a box levitate.

Edith said she had a headache develop while driving with Peter to their appointment with me and this headache continued to worsen during the interview. I suspected that dark forces were doing their usual, namely causing the patient to get lost or get sick, so they, the dark forces, won't be discovered and eliminated.

Peter's interview also made references to extraterrestrial implants. He said that in 1994 he had a lucid out-of-body dream wherein he found himself sitting on a chair seeing instruments above him. He was being told that an implant was being placed in his head. He also said that he could see energy beings and that he felt like he had a shield of energy all around him.

I began the induction in a very orderly fashion, and as I did, Edith began to clutch her head and move all over the couch in pain from the headache, which worsened as soon as we started the induction. I placed my crucifix on her forehead and told her that her headaches will cease, and she will relax and feel good. I have taken this action many times with patients and have found that it is the best defense against the dark forces. Edith's pain stopped within thirty seconds. I was fortunate in that I soon found myself speaking to a valid Spirit Guide within each of them. Both Spirit Guides agreed that Edith had many dark force entities, Peter had three, and both groups of dark forces included powerful ones. At this moment an evil smile came over Edith, and she began to laugh in an ominous fashion. I decided to not waste any time and immediately conducted an exorcism which removed all the dark forces attached directly to both patients.

I now asked the Spirit Guides to check for frequencies of further foreign energy that may be present. When asked about the presence of Earthbound spirits, the two Spirit Guides agreed that Edith had six Earthbound spirits, but Peter had none. They also agreed that Edith's Earthbound spirits were draining energy from her but were not contributing to her problems, except for one, who was found to have a powerful dark force attachment. A second exorcism removed this powerful dark force. Following this, I helped all the Earthbound spirits get to the Light.

We then turned our attention towards detecting any soul fragments that might be attached and found that Edith was overwhelmed with close to a thousand of them, all of whom have fragmented from their respective souls due to the trauma of an alien abduction (once again we are seeing soul fragments being drawn to an individual who has had similar negative experiences.) It became obvious that negative and hostile comments were being directed toward Edith from many of the soul fragments, and that's when Peter's Spirit Guide noticed that a large dark cloud accompanied the soul fragments. Usually these dark clouds are full of dark forces and powerful dark forces that are hiding. A third successful exorcism was called into place, a soul retrieval was then carried out, and all the fragments were returned to their original souls, including one that was attached to Peter.

Following the soul retrieval, Edith's Spirit Guide discovered two entities that said they were Earthbound spirits and were her family from a past life and had made a contract with Edith in the afterlife so as to be able to join her in this lifetime. Both Spirit Guides instantly spoke out in a loud voice, saying, "They are lying... they are dark forces!" A fourth exorcism was immediately performed removing both dark forces.

Both Spirit Guides saw that Edith and Peter had extraterrestrials present along with implants. I asked to speak to the leader of the extraterrestrials who was attached to Edith. He identified himself as 'Morac,' a Reptilian, who said, "They are like family... I own them. We have abducted them many times starting when they were babies."

I asked many questions and was told that yes, they did experiments on Edith and Peter, took eggs and semen, and placed many implants within them. According to the Spirit Guides, Edith has eight implants and Peter, five. Usually the leader of the aliens attaches to the host, and the remaining extraterrestrials hover nearby. Edith had three Reptilians including Morac, the attached leader. Peter, on the other hand, had an attached extraterrestrial leader and one other extraterrestrial, both of whom were from an insectoid species who were helping the Reptilians. Both Edith and Peter were the victims of the Reptilians who did the abductions and placed the implants; however, both species were extremely evil, and I was not about to attempt to negotiate their removal of implants and their departure, so I went ahead with my fifth exorcism and asked for extra help from all the Archangels, as many Master Spirits as we could get to help,

St. Germain, and finally, Jesus. The battle raged for a short time and finally both Spirit Guides confirmed that St. Michael the Archangel had taken all the extraterrestrials and their implants to that special place in the Light where he takes them.

Edith and Peter's souls were found to be fragmented from the many abductions, so a soul retrieval was performed, and they now have complete souls and are much less vulnerable to entity infestation. The patients were instructed in God Light visualization and affirmations so as to maintain their protective state. Both patients were awakened from their hypnotic altered state feeling much lighter, happier, more relaxed, more positive and loving, and full of renewed energy.

A FATHER'S LOVE

A patient from Chicago that I had seen previously called me about his thirteen-year-old son, Billy. It seems that Billy became exceptionally emotional for the past several years with occasional outbursts. His father was concerned because Billy was becoming progressively more depressed and saddened over simple things and had very little self-confidence. His father's concern heightened over the past year when Billy began talking about killing himself.

Billy's father's Spirit Guide had been exceptionally helpful, so I suggested a dual hypnosis using both Billy and his father. It was obvious that dark forces were involved, so hypnotizing both Billy and his father together would double my chance of getting to a Spirit Guide. This was a good decision, as I was only able to get to the father's Spirit Guide, who informed me that Billy's father had five dark force entities, but his son Billy had a great many. The exorcism lasted over thirty minutes, as it was necessary for me to invoke the help of all the Archangels, available Master Spirits, and finally, our savior Jesus Christ. The father's Spirit Guide confirmed that all dark force entities had been taken to the Light; however, the Spirit Guide seemed overwhelmed and did not return. I was able to make contact with a second Spirit Guide from the father, who had very little experience with detecting the frequency of foreign energy. I then asked for a third Spirit Guide, who was able to continue the entity releasement and said that the son, Billy, had four Earthbound spirits. While I was interviewing the Earthbound spirits, the father's Spirit Guide mentioned that he saw darkness within one of these Earthbound spirits and then yelled out, "He's a powerful dark force entity pretending to be an Earthbound spirit!"

I quickly conducted another exorcism and went back to interviewing the remaining Earthbound spirit, who was very helpful and informed me that the dark force pretender was responsible for the heavy emotions and the suicidal tendency which resulted from very dark thoughts. This exceptionally observant Earthbound spirit also said that Billy's negative emotions and poor self-confidence were the result of many years of being told he was stupid by his mother and by other students.

After helping the remaining Earthbound spirits get to the Light, I uncovered the fact that Billy had been fragmented for quite some time. Following completion of a successful soul retrieval, Billy once again became a complete soul. At this time his father's Spirit Guide confirmed that Billy and his father were now free of foreign energy. I followed with my dissertation on God Light visualization and affirmation and powerful suggestions to the subconscious mind and wrapped up the session. During a follow up phone call many months later, I was told that Billy had improved on all fronts.

DUAL HYPNOSIS USING AN ASSISTANT

THE HEALER WHO WAS AN ABDUCTEE

George was a 27-year-old patient who was only able to fly in from New Orleans for one appointment. His concerns centered on several issues, including health problems, fear stemming from being rescued from a house fire when he was one year old, a need to know if he had ever been molested, and a need to know if he had ever been abducted by aliens. He also felt that something was holding him back from being successful, and he said that knowing his life's purpose or lesson for this life would be exceptionally helpful. George was also very concerned about when he would meet his wife-to-be, the woman of his dreams. When will this part of his life begin?

My Higher Self told me that it would make more sense to do an initial dual hypnosis with my assistant and guarantee a successful outcome for the session, since I had only one appointment to work with. Following hypnotic induction and contact with my assistant's Spirit Guide, permission was obtained from the patient to check for and remove foreign energy. The Spirit Guide identified one dark force entity, two Earthbound spirits, and several soul fragments. Once the exorcism was completed I interrogated the Earthbound spirits, the first of whom was a female who had been with the patient for many lifetimes. She said she had been his lover, his sister, and other individuals who had been close to him in all those lifetimes. The purpose of her joining him was because she loved him and wanted to protect him. This Earthbound spirit said that her mission was to help people by bringing them Light and understanding and mentioned that George has had lifetimes on other planets. She also felt that George had a concern about being molested because both she and he had been molested by a cousin in the same past lifetime. She was four years old at the time, and he was three. This Earthbound spirit then said that George had not been molested in this present lifetime; however his sister was fondled by a young boy.

The second Earthbound spirit had been with the patient for four years, and his purpose was to learn from the patient. Neither of the two Earthbound spirits had health issues that contributed to George's health problems. Both of these Earthbound spirits readily agreed to go to the Light, so I helped them do so and wished them Godspeed. Once a soul retrieval was performed for the several soul fragments who had not contributed to George's problems, the patient was pronounced free of foreign energy and instructed on God Light visualizations and affirmations. Also, George was found to be a complete soul which had not been fragmented.

I now asked my assistant's Spirit Guide about George's strong feelings that he may have been abducted by aliens. George had listened to tapes recording his mother's hypnosis sessions, which indicated that his mother, sister, and grandfather, had all been abducted. Also, he had become very disturbed as a toddler when he saw a picture of a Gray alien and told his mother that he had been chased by them down some sort of a tunnel.

The Spirit Guide replied, "Yes, George has had three alien abductions in this lifetime, but no aliens or implants remain." He continued, "George has been wounded as a healer in several past lifetimes. He is very sensitive and is quite empathetic. He was able to heal others by understanding. His lesson is to help others by caring and teaching. George needs to release guilt, open his heart, and be grateful. His health problem came from a compromised immune system; he needs to laugh more, and this will definitely improve his immune system. Finally, he is to be ready for love to come, and it will come."

The patient notified me a few weeks later to say that he was very much improved and had a much more positive outlook on life.

DUAL HYPNOSIS IS A PROBLEM FOR DARK FORCES

Dark forces are able to keep one's Spirit Guide from coming forth and are often able to prevent that person from being able to regress, but they have a definite problem interfering with dual hypnosis, which utilizes a second person's Spirit Guide during the hypnotic session. Jeffrey, a 48-year-old real estate agent from California, is one of hundreds of patients who were able to skirt the dark force influence and get to the bottom of his problem by using dual hypnosis. Jeffrey came to see me so as to alleviate anxiety accompanied by panic attacks, depression, fear of intimacy, and a fear of engaging people on a social level, especially people he's unfamiliar with, causing him to stutter and become very nauseated.

An important part of his history stood out like a neon sign. At a very young age Jeffrey was molested by a teenaged male cousin who was watching him while his family went to a graduation ceremony. He was embarrassed and afraid to say anything to his family or anyone else.

Jeffrey easily slipped into deep hypnosis, but difficulties soon began when I could not get to a Spirit Guide or regress him. I have seen this situation all too often and immediately suspected a dark force interference. When I incur such circumstances I do not waste valuable time under deep hypnosis but rather take an hour or more to infuse powerful positive suggestions and protective measures firmly into the patient's subconscious mind. After waking the patient from hypnosis I explained that dark forces are definitely the cause of this situation and would highly recommend a second appointment for dual hypnosis using my assistant. I emphasized that this follow up appointment would be 100% successful in removing all entities and getting to and analyzing the cause of his issues. After explaining the above to Jeffrey, he fully understood and eagerly agreed to return for a dual hypnosis session.

Several days later a dual hypnosis was performed, and a lengthy exorcism was carried out to remove many dark forces, including powerful ones. Seven Earthbound spirits who had not contributed to Jeffrey's issues were happy to go to the Light. As usual, the emotions from a person who has been molested were powerful enough to act as a magnet and attract fragments of other people's souls who had similar experiences. Four such soul fragments were found and returned to their original souls by performing a soul retrieval. Jeffrey was now pronounced free of foreign energy.

My assistant's Spirit Guide now weighed in on Jeffrey's problems and said, "His intimacy problem stems from his molestation. He is sad and lonely and thinks his feelings are not important. He also feels guilty and dirty at the same time and carries much anger for his cousin and his parents for bringing him to his home. He needs to have unconditional love for himself and reach deeply within his heart for forgiveness for both his parents and his cousin. Once he does these things, he will be able to give and receive love and no longer feel guilt, anxiety, or depression."

I followed with a soul retrieval for his many missing soul fragments, making him once again a complete soul and thus less vulnerable to entity attachment. We ended the session with him promising himself and me that he will make it a point to do his God Light visualizations and affirmations as we have discussed to maintain protection. Follow up some time later found Jeffrey to be much happier with improvement across the board, especially in his love life.

MOTIVATION MAY COME WITH A PRICE

This extremely intelligent 51-year-old woman from Atlantic City, New Jersey, presented with excessive anxiety, panic attacks, and depression, which began three years earlier, after she had put a lot of time and creative energy into designing, developing, and running a successful business. The patient says she has not been happy for the past four years, during which time she has also had an excessive amount of skin rashes. She thinks that these feelings have sabotaged her marriage and her sex life. She then relayed the occurrence of several unusual behaviors that she has displayed over the past several years that were not like her. These included being calmer while traveling in the mid-west; having an anxiety attack, a bloody nose, and fainting following a commercial airline takeoff; feeling very comfortable in a casino; having an overwhelming urge to go to gun clubs; and craving sausage pizza in spite of being on a wheat-free diet.

My hypnotic induction elicited all the signs of dark forces being present. I was unable to regress the patient or have a Spirit Guide come forward. The patient described herself being immersed in complete blackness when she felt something pushing on her head. Soon the pressure became pain that involved the top and sides of her head. When this occurred I touched her head with the crucifix and told her that I was placing a God Light helmet on her head. The pain immediately ceased. I now decided to call this dark force out into the open. As I did so, the patient felt something pushing her eyes open, ending the session.

The patient returned for a dual hypnosis with my assistant. The session revealed a powerful dark force who was removed by exorcism and one Earthbound spirit by the name of *Red*, who joined the patient approximately six years ago. This man was quite intelligent and said that he died in his nineties in 1923. He was a motivational and inspirational orator and also an inventor who loved to make things work better. He also loved to play poker, ate sausage pizza, and always carried a gun. When I asked about his purpose in attaching to the patient, his response was, "To get her going, personally and in business."

My assistant's Spirit Guide now filled in the spaces, saying, "Red had been a tremendous help in getting the patient's business up and running. He would inspire and motivate her in many ways, so much so that she had very little time for herself, causing her unbearable anxiety. The amount of work going into business was enabling her to feel successful but overwhelmed and sometimes not being able to think straight. She was beginning to feel as if she was a workhorse on autopilot and therefore not very attractive. This situation has greatly contributed to her anxiety, which has led to marriage problems and constant skin rashes." Red was happy to go to the Light, and a soul retrieval was performed to retrieve the many fragments of the patient's soul which had split away due to this excessive traumatic stress. No past lifetimes contributed to her depression. The patient was now instructed in God Light protection.

A follow up over two years later revealed an extremely happy patient with very few issues or marriage problems. The patient's rashes ceased to exist almost immediately after our session, and her interest in guns and casinos has dwindled. All in all, she is much happier and very grateful.

Chapter 15

REMOTE ENTITY RELEASEMENT

What I call "remote entity releasement" is similar to Dr. Baldwin's *remote spirit releasement.* It is performed in the office for a patient who is not physically present by either using the Spirit Guide of a friend or a relative who comes into the office on behalf of the patient who was unable to come in personally, or by using my assistant's Spirit Guide. I use the term "remote patient" to refer to the person being treated, who is absent, and the term "office patient" for the person I am seeing in my office for the benefit of the remote patient. Thus, the office patient or my assistant acts as an intermediary for the remote patient, who is usually a long distance from my office, often from different states or even foreign countries. This remote form of entity releasement differs from Dr. Baldwin's remote spirit releasement in that I use the intermediary's Spirit Guide to monitor the session, confirm the presence of entities, and assist me in releasing them. The U.S. government has been researching and successfully performing remote viewing, which is considered a non-local connection. I agree with Dr. Baldwin that this method of depossession, performed remotely, is another form of a non-local connection.

People diagnosed as having various forms of mental disorders, including schizophrenia, have requested remote entity releasement since they are unable to travel to see me. Many of them heard voices or felt something touching them. Some maintained anger, fear, and frustration, and many were suicidal. All of these cases were shown to have massive numbers of foreign energy attachments, which almost always included large numbers of dark forces and powerful dark forces. Patients who are remote are informed of protective measures, or these protections are remotely sent to them by the friend or loved one acting as the intermediary. Loved ones immediately noticed changes for the good, as did the patients themselves.

People diagnosed with physical ailments have also seen improvements. A good example of this was a young man with a diagnosis of schizophrenia and a brain tumor. My assistant's Spirit Guide discovered and removed an extraterrestrial implant and predicted improvement of both conditions. During a follow up one month later, I was told that the young man looks better, eats better, and doesn't appear to be in a daze any more. A follow up several months later revealed that a recent MRI had shown that the brain tumor is getting smaller.

REMOTE ENTITY RELEASEMENT USING AN ASSISTANT

LOSING LOVE HURTS DEEPLY

A remote entity releasement session was scheduled for Herbert, a 36-year-old man from the state of Washington who has had a severe form of depression for many years. He is on medication and sees a therapist routinely but still cannot hold down a job due to his inability to concentrate on what needs to be done and follow through with what's needed. He is quite fearful and has nothing positive to say about himself. This rather severe condition has kept him at home with his parents, who have asked me to perform a remote entity releasement on their son, who was aware of when the session would take place.

The remote session began with my assistant's Spirit Guide requesting and obtaining permission from Herbert's Higher Self. His foreign energy included six or more dark forces, who, according to the Spirit Guide, appeared to be coming and going. I immediately conducted the exorcism, and all dark force entities that were present were taken to the Light and confirmed to be there. The only foreign energy remaining was a soul fragment from a living teenaged drug addict, who fragmented when he almost died of a drug overdose. According to my assistant's Spirit Guide, the teenager is still an addict, but this soul fragment does not share in the addictive tendency. A soul retrieval was carried out.

My assistant's Spirit Guide now said, "Herbert has undergone a fragmentation of his own soul from a traumatic incident which was really a loss. I now hear the name Beverly; she is the cause of the sense of loss that makes Herbert feel alone. She encouraged him to be happy, and now she's gone. This makes him feel that no one understands how he feels and puts thoughts in his head like, what's the use in trying to be happy? It's easier to be depressed." Herbert now underwent a soul retrieval, was found to have no past lifetimes contributing to his depression, and finally was sent Light and love by my assistant's Spirit Guide.

When I gave a report to Herbert's parents, they told me that Beverly was the love of his life who left him a few years ago. Several weeks later I received a follow up call on Herbert from his parents. They said they saw a remarkable, visible improvement in him. He feels lighter and is very chipper and brighter and laughs much more than ever before. He even volunteered that he felt really good the day of the session, something he has not said in quite a while. He is continuing to go to his therapist to work though his heartbreak and other depressive issues. As per my instruction his parents are sending him white God Light protection often, since he doesn't believe in anything spiritual. Hopefully they can convince him to come in for an appointment.

IMPLANTS CAN ATTRACT DARK FORCES

This fifty-eight-year-old insurance agent from Oregon came to me with complaints of chronic migraine headaches, insomnia, and vascular issues. His history included seeing a face with dark eyes at night and feeling something on his leg that seemed to leave a mark. This made me immediately suspicious of the presence of dark forces. The patient easily attained deep hypnosis but would not regress nor allow a Spirit Guide to come forth. I was now sure we were dealing with dark forces and suggested that I conduct a remote entity releasement on him since he had to return home that evening.

My assistant and I performed a remote releasement of entities two weeks later and discovered a large number of dark forces. In addition to the dark forces, several Reptilian extraterrestrials and two implants, one in his neck and one in his leg, were identified. The dark force entities, extraterrestrials, and the two implants were taken to the special place in the Light that St. Michael the Archangel takes them. No past life events were contributory, and the patient has not been fragmented. My assistant's Spirit Guide sent the patient protective God Light and then commented that I should be aware that dark forces are usually attracted by–and are drawn to–implants that are left by extraterrestrials. The patient notified me several months later that his insomnia and migraine headaches have greatly improved.

PSYCHIC ABILITIES CAN BE A DOUBLE-EDGED SWORD

The following case is yet another example of a patient having a problem due to multiple causes. Such examples clearly show the necessity of including entity releasement in a past life regression therapy session. The regression therapist is not there to just take the patient into past lifetimes; he's there to cure the patient.

I received a call from Atlanta, Georgia, from the uncle of a twenty-eight-year-old woman who had psychic abilities and was often ill, having massive mood swings whereupon she would become quite depressed to the point of being suicidal. She occasionally would cut herself during some of those episodes. Her husband was unsuccessful at trying to help her feel better. I told the uncle that we would be glad to do a remote entity releasement and to please let the patient and her husband know when the session will take place and to expect a call shortly following the session.

My assistant and I carried out a remote session six days later. Following hypnotic induction of my assistant, her Spirit Guide was able to locate and obtain permission from the patient's Higher Self to remove foreign energy. When I asked about the presence of foreign energy, I heard a resounding, "Yes!" We removed many dark force entities and three soul fragments, all of which were contributing to the patient's problem. In addition, one of the soul fragments also had psychic abilities that added to those of the patient, causing the patient's family to consider her abilities evil.

Following removal of all attached entities and a soul retrieval for the patient who was found to have a fragmented soul, my assistant's Spirit Guide, as usual, came up with prudent and profound insights regarding the patient's problem and weighed in on the situation, saying, "The patient has a heavy load to carry, a feeling of imbalance from a past lifetime, which keeps her feeling ill and makes her a magnet for attracting dark force entities and troubled soul fragments, which have continued to affect her adversely. The patient had psychic abilities in several past lifetimes. One of those lifetimes resulted in her being burned at the stake as a witch. This very emotional and traumatic death memory has imprinted a powerful misbelief in her subconscious mind, namely that being psychic means something is wrong with you and you can die because of this. This kind of thinking kept the patient feeling unworthy and living in fear. The dark force entities, as usual, took advantage of the situation by encouraging and magnifying the negativity to the point of making the patient suicidal." Following this astute evaluation, the Guide then sent the patient Light, love, and blessings.

Soon after the session came to a close, I called the patient's uncle and gave him a detailed report on the remote entity releasement session and told him that protection from further entity infestation could be possible by having his niece carry out God Light visualizations and affirmations, which I described in detail. In addition, I emphasized that if she doesn't do this consistently, either he or her husband can do it for her and at the same time send her this God Light. This affirmation lets entities and especially dark forces know where you stand and that you are the captain of your soul and not open to uninvited attachments.

I received a call from the patient's uncle approximately six weeks after the session. He told me that his niece had been terribly afflicted for years but now has improved tremendously, and he has never seen her look better.

REMOTE ENTITY RELEASEMENT USING A PATIENT'S SPIRIT GUIDE

It is amazing how fast the word gets out regarding something that will enable one to help someone he or she loves. I have had a surprising number of patients who had appointments tell me that a loved one at home requested that I also perform a remote entity releasement on him as well. They probably heard me mention doing remote entity releasements on a patient's loved one during a patient's session, from other patients, or from radio interviews. Entity infestation is so common that most people who are enlightened and aware of the existence of such entities feel obligated to clean the slate, not only on themselves but on those they love.

All I require during such sessions is a valid and experienced Spirit Guide who comes forth when requested during the patient's session. Once the patient's Spirit Guide is on board, we are able to accomplish a tremendous amount of good. This includes getting to the cause of the patient's issues by interrogating and then removing foreign energy, reviewing past life memories that have contributed to these issues, healing the patient's soul if it is fragmented, and giving instructions on protection and prevention.

If the patient has a distant friend or loved one who requests that I utilize the patient's Spirit Guide to help him as well, I then ask the patient's Spirit Guide to please accomplish this and start by getting permission from the remote person's Higher Self. I have had many such requests to remotely help a patient's lover, spouse, child, sibling, parent, and friend, and the feedback from such sessions is most gratifying. The following case is quite interesting and serves as a typical example of this method of remotely removing entities using the patient who is seeing me as an intermediary.

HOW TO IMPROVE YOUR SEX LIFE

Sharon is a 28-year-old woman from Minneapolis who came to see me because of relationship problems with her fiancé, William. Sharon and William are very much in love and want to get married, however Sharon is becoming progressively more concerned about their sex life, which has left her unfulfilled. William seems to enjoy 'quickies' and is not concerned with Sharon's pleasure or whether she has been satisfied.

Sharon and William both feel that he may have foreign energy attachments that may be causing this behavior and were wondering if I could depossess him remotely since he could not accompany her on this trip. I informed the patient that we need a good Spirit Guide to come forth to accomplish this. Proceeding with the induction, Sharon entered deep hypnosis and called forth her Spirit Guide, who was very helpful by immediately pronouncing Sharon free of foreign energy and stating that her soul has not been fragmented, and that she has no past lives that have contributed to this particular problem.

We then asked Sharon's Spirit Guide if he could locate her fiancé, William, and receive permission from his Higher Self to remove entities. This permission was given, thus making William a remote patient. According to the Spirit Guide, William definitely had foreign energy present. One powerful dark force was identified, and a full exorcism was successfully conducted and completed, thus removing this powerful dark force and having him taken to that special place in the Light that St. Michael the Archangel takes him. Three male Earthbound spirits were found to be attached to William. The first one had several lifetimes with William and had very interesting things to say about making love to a woman. This Earthbound spirit said that he was deformed when he was born into his prior lifetime and therefore visited brothels to satisfy his sexual urges. He said he was more comfortable making love quickly so as not to expose his deformity any longer than necessary and really was not concerned about satisfying the woman.

The second Earthbound spirit was aggressive to the point of being hostile. I instantly suspected and quickly confirmed the presence of four dark forces that were attached to him. A second exorcism was successfully carried out, leaving this Earthbound spirit to now exhibit his own personality which I felt was still rather obnoxious. His comment was that when he was alive, he was very apathetic when making love, and he thought that this made him a good lover. He then said, "I feel like William, and he is now just like me. We both have great apathy when it comes to making love."

The third Earthbound spirit had a congenital heart defect while he was alive and died suddenly while making love at age 21. He felt that William should hurry when making love because if you drag it on, you may get a heart attack. I was able to convince all three Earthbound spirits to go to the Light and helped them to do so. I then wished them Godspeed.

The remaining foreign energy infesting William consisted of several soul fragments, two of which were influencing William's lovemaking techniques. The first such soul fragment separated from his soul some three hundred years ago due to his being beaten as a slave at age sixteen. He did not know anything about lovemaking and felt entirely embarrassed about the subject of making love.

The second soul fragment causing problems separated from his soul when he was forty years old in this present lifetime. The trauma responsible for his soul fragmentation was from being shot by a prostitute. At the time, he was doing what he enjoyed the most, sadomasochistic sex, bondage, autoerotic asphyxia, and deriving pleasure from his causing pain in a female partner. He said he often gave William such thoughts.

A soul retrieval for all soul fragments attached to William was carried out so that the soul fragments were returned safely to their original souls. The Spirit Guide concluded the session by saying that Sharon and William had fifteen lifetimes together, five of which they shared as lovers. None of these lifetimes were related to the problems that Sharon and William are presently having. William himself has been fragmented from various traumatic episodes in his lifetime. We then accomplished a soul retrieval for William, making him once again a complete soul and less vulnerable to future entity attachment. The Guide now said that their sex life will now improve slowly but steadily. I followed with instructions for Sharon to routinely carry out God Light visualizations and affirmations for herself and William and also to have William routinely do this. This is one of my more recent cases, just prior to the publishing of this book. As such, I do not have a follow up as yet; however, I am very sure that Sharon and William's sex life will be very much improved.

Chapter 16

THE SOLEMN RITE OF EXORCISM

DEFINITION

The definition of exorcism, according to the catechism of the Catholic Church, is: "When the Church asks publicly and authoritatively in the name of Jesus Christ that a person or object be protected against the power of the Evil One and withdrawn from his dominion, it is called exorcism."[10]

NEW GUIDELINES

The Vatican's newest guidelines on exorcism were presented during a news conference at the Vatican on January 26, 1999. These 1999 guidelines updated the previous set that was written in the year 1614. This original and traditional Rite of Exorcism, written in Latin, is allowed as an option. The new guideline titled, *Of Exorcism and Certain Supplications*, is used in the ritual along with prayers, blessings, and invocations. An assumption is made that an individual who is possessed still has his free will even though his physical body may

---

10 Fr. Gabriele Amorth. *An Exorcist Tells His Story*. San Francisco: Ignatius Press, 1999, p. 43.

be controlled by a demon. Exorcisms are a solemn rite that can only be performed by an ordained priest or higher prelate and must have the permission of the local bishop and a prior medical examination to rule out mental or physical illness. Signs of possible demonic possession of a person, according to the Roman Ritual, include supernatural strength and abilities, speaking languages unknown to him, violent reaction to religious objects, knowing things he shouldn't know, and profuse blasphemy.

NEED FOR MORE EXORCISTS

In the fall of 2010, the nation's Roman Catholic bishops held a two day conference in Baltimore, Maryland, that was designed to train priests on how to conduct exorcisms. According to the Catholic news service, more than fifty bishops and sixty priests signed up for the conference. The organizer of the conference, Bishop Thomas Paprocki, said that only a very small number of American priests have enough training and knowledge to perform exorcisms, which are performed only rarely; however, in the last several years this small number of adequately trained clergy has been overwhelmed with requests to evaluate parishioners who claim to be possessed. No one seems to know why there are more people seeking the rite of exorcism. Some have suggested that more Americans are looking to spirituality rather than organized religion; others are saying that many Catholic immigrants in America have come from countries where exorcism is more accepted. My own thought regarding this increased need for exorcism is that the battle between good and evil is escalating, and the dark forces are pouring it on wherever possible.

Cardinal Stanislow Dziwisz, the private secretary of Pope John Paul II, revealed that even Pope John Paul had performed an exorcism on a woman who was brought to the Vatican with obvious signs of what appeared to be demonic possession. I am sure that many Catholics are unaware that their own sacrament of baptism contained a minor form of exorcism that included prayers that renounced Satan and sought freedom from original sin.

For those who are extremely interested in the history of spirit possession and exorcism, I highly recommend Dr. William Baldwin's classic book, *Spirit Releasement Therapy.* In his book Dr. Baldwin presents an excellent comprehensive review of the historical accounts of possession and exorcism.

THANK GOD FOR SPIRIT GUIDES

I must say that I am grateful to have confirmation that the entity has arrived at a specified destination following releasement, a task that is superbly carried out by a valid and helpful Spirit Guide. On the positive side, I must also say that the Catholic Church is telling us that evil is very real and exists in the form of non-physical, non-human demonic entities who can attach to humans and affect them greatly in an adverse way. And yes, I find it very rewarding to hear comments from those in the hierarchy of the Catholic Church such as the one made during an interview with a newspaper reporter prior to the 2010 exorcism training conference. One of the speakers at the conference, Cardinal Daniel DiNardo, Archbishop of Galveston-Houston, Texas, said, "For the longest time, we in the United States may not have been as much attuned to some of the spiritual aspects of evil because we have become so much attached to what would be either physical or psychological explanation for certain phenomena... We may have forgotten that there is a spiritual dimension to people."[11]

---

11 Zoll, Rachel. "Catholic Bishops Say More Exorcists are Needed," *Associated Press*, November 13, 2010, Las Vegas Review Journal.

Chapter 17

WHAT'S MISSING IN MEDICINE

THE ENDLESS BATTLE

It has become obvious to me that the battle of good versus evil is looming large in the world today. School shootings have occurred often enough that most schools now have a protocol for such incidents. We must not forget the Scandinavian man who, in a crazed frenzy, killed 77 people in Norway in July of 2011, including a great number of children. The following year, a well-respected American soldier supposedly went over the edge and massacred seventeen Afghanistan civilians, including several children, as they slept.

I am convinced that when many powerful dark force entities attach to people, they are able to have an unbelievable influence over them and have them truly do their bidding. This form of attachment can easily be called a full possession. The cases mentioned in the prior paragraph fall into that demonic category, as does another, which occurred while I was writing this chapter. The July 20, 2012, news referred to it as the "Aurora Massacre," wherein a so-called madman stepped into a nighttime showing of a new Batman movie in Aurora, Colorado, and opened fire, killing twelve and injuring fifty eight men, women, and children. The killer identified himself as "The Joker," a vengeful villain in Batman movies and comics. The carnage would have risen dramatically had the gunman's assault rifle not jammed. This madman was a relatively normal neuroscience student who started to have danger signs and eventually was seen by a psychiatrist and diagnosed as having schizophrenia.

Governments, legal systems, and medical evaluations struggle to come up with the motive for such unexpected and hideous actions on the part of these mostly adult human beings who are not affiliated with any terrorist organization and who were mostly quite normal prior to the incident.

The news has also had many stories of children from age five to the early teens who suddenly became dangerous and destructive and so out of control that they had to be handcuffed or restrained in other ways so they wouldn't hurt themselves or others or destroy property. One ten-year-old even brandished a gun. Families often say, "I don't understand; he was always so nice." I don't claim to be an expert by any stretch of the imagination, but I have witnessed adults and children who had become somewhat demonic return to normal following a depossession which removed many dark force entities and sometimes powerful dark forces.

My experience with Comprehensive Hypnoregression sessions has shown that once a person dies and enters the Light, he knows who he is, an eternal being that has passed through an incarnation cycle and is now home where he started from. In the Light the soul becomes focused on lessons that it needed to learn and karma it needed to balance in that lifetime. Earthly thoughts regarding specific events in that lifetime now take a back seat to what is really important, namely spiritual matters.

A soul may decline going to the Light for many reasons. I believe that one of these reasons is due to the presence of powerful dark forces or a large number of dark forces persuading a person's soul to decline going to the Light before, during, and following the death experience. This soul will then remain in the lower astral plane as an Earthbound spirit with these dark attachments and have the same thoughts, feelings, desires, addictions, and so on, that it did when it was alive and in a body; but because of the dark force influence, this Earthbound spirit will have a dark side which can cause an extreme amount of negative influence when the Earthbound spirit decides to attach to a human being.

If a terrorist leader was killed while carrying out his well-planned mission of terror, he most likely would still feel a need to do so as an Earthbound spirit in the lower astral plane. I feel that this scenario applies to the Jet Blue commercial airline flight that turned into a nightmare for the passengers on March 27, 2012. The airline captain, a very responsible and loving family man, began acting strangely in the cockpit, pushing buttons and grabbing the throttle, causing the copilot to devise a reason for the captain to leave the cockpit and then lock him out. The captain returned and began banging and kicking on the door, ranting and raving about bombs and al Qaida, and was finally restrained by passengers until an emergency landing was accomplished.

I think it is very possible that such an Earthbound spirit, with its dark force attachments, decided to attach to that Jet Blue commercial pilot for the purpose of crashing the airplane. I feel that the uncontrollable, bizarre behavior of that pilot was due to a tug of war between his true self and a determined Earthbound spirit with a terrorist agenda and a powerful dark force influence. At that time, I felt that if in the future a commercial airline pilot exhibits a similar, bizarre behavior, I will know that I am right.

Several years have elapsed since that incident occurred, and now the news broadcasts are brimming over with news flashes regarding another commercial airliner that crashed in the French Alps, killing 150 people. The information from one of the black boxes seemed to indicate that the captain left the cockpit, most likely to use the restroom, and he was locked out of the cockpit by the copilot. The black box picked up pounding noises and shouting which came from the captain, attempting to get back into the cockpit. The copilot obviously would not unlock the cockpit door, and the plane began to descend from 38,000 feet at more than 3,000 feet per minute. One of the black boxes indicated that the copilot accelerated the descent several times. We were later told that the altitude had been reset at 100 feet by the copilot. The plane crashed into the mountains, killing all aboard. Investigators later found that the copilot had been seen by a doctor who wrote a note saying he was unfit to fly because of a mental disorder. He had also been considered to be suicidal at one time.

If a person is very depressed or has mental problems making him suicidal, this would usually be carried out in a more private manner and not like a terrorist suicide bomber. Based on my extensive experience with entities attached to patients, I strongly feel that my theory involving the possession of a commercial airline captain or copilot by a terrorist Earthbound spirit is quite possible in that it enables this Earthbound spirit to carry out these extremely evil deeds through its host.

STRESS AND THE POWER OF EMOTIONS

It is a known fact that psychological stress can cause anxiety and depression which, according to research, will lower a person's immune response (protection from disease). Most people are aware of the fact that an impaired immune response could lead to various types of illness; however, many of them do not realize that these illnesses include different forms of virus-associated cancers, such as Kaposi Sarcoma and certain lymphomas. Research has shown that the effects of stress on the immune system may also affect the growth of some tumors.

Recent research by an international group of 440 scientists has led them to the conclusion that "junk DNA," which composes 98% of the DNA, actually serves as a "switch" that can turn genes on and off. This would explain why individuals who are predisposed to certain diseases get them, while others do not. Vulnerability to certain cancers and other diseases may or may not develop, depending on the stimulus that affects the "switches." The human genome is thought to contain at least four million of these switches.

One researcher named John Stamatoyannopoulos was quoted as saying, "The whole way that we look at the genetic basis of disease is going to change."[12] A lot more research needs to be carried out so as to determine the function of each of these switches. According to another researcher, Evan Birney, "It's going to take this century to fill in all the details."[13] In my opinion, psychological stress will be found to be an important environmental factor that can stimulate these "switches," which will in turn switch on the "bad gene" and allow the cancer or other diseases to surface.

So, how does one become psychologically stressed? It all starts with a negative thought, which brings about a negative emotion, which can be a strong reaction to a situation that goes beyond one's coping capabilities. This is especially true if the negative thought or emotion causes an emotional past life memory to surface and exacerbate the situation. Life on Earth is not easy, so such reactions can easily become a chronic pattern of negativity, followed by negative emotions, with physiologic ramifications resulting in the persistent activation of the hypothalamic-pituitary-adrenal hormonal axis, which leads to anxiety, depression, increased heart rate, increased blood pressure, increased blood sugar, and chronic suppression of the immune system. These chronic negative reactions will often rev up one's negative emotions to the degree that will make him more vulnerable to dark force attachment and thus worsen the person's condition and possibly make him suicidal. Also, the law of attraction may be put into play, and this most unfortunate person would draw even more negativity to himself.

Following an investigation of a patient's foreign energy and the influence it has upon his emotional or physical problem, I will then

---

12 "DNA Switches: A New Insight into Genes." The Week, 21 Sept. 2012: 21.
13 Ibid: 21.

ask the patient's Spirit Guide if any present, future, or past life events are the emotional cause of the problem or have at least contributed heavily to it. If so, I request that the Spirit Guide take the patient back to those events. You may question my referring to the cause of these problems as being emotional. I do so because man is an emotional being. Every action that he carries out is involved with one emotion or another. The human condition by its very nature is immersed in emotions of all kinds, both positive and negative, and everything in between. The cases that have been presented easily demonstrate why people need to seek Comprehensive Hypnoregression Therapy for issues that are ongoing and contribute daily to the stockpiles of negative emotions that weigh heavily upon their shoulders. Emotions cannot be ignored, especially in medicine.

PROMINENT MEMORIES

Memories stored in the subconscious mind become prominent because of the emotions they have evoked in the patient in that particular lifetime. Prominent emotional memories are the ones that stand out and are able to literally cripple people mentally, physically, and spiritually once they are brought to the forefront of the subconscious mind. The effect of such negative programming of the conscious mind by this very emotional subconscious memory is suffering, with no conscious knowledge of why. These prominent subconscious memories are literally lifted up from the depths of the subconscious and brought forward. This metamorphosis of a past memory occurs when a person, place, or thing in a person's present life becomes a catalyst, a kind of déjà vu that triggers and ignites the powerful emotions that accompanied a long-forgotten memory. This memory is thus maneuvered into a unique position within the subconscious, so it is now able to evoke extreme negative emotions within the conscious mind.

THE CONSCIOUS OBSERVER

The beauty of the hypnotic state is that the conscious mind is fully awake and aware of everything that's happening while the therapist brings up the subconscious mind and all its long forgotten memories. The conscious mind is now able to observe from a safe distance and digest what the subconscious brings forth and is thus able to make rational judgments and decisions in regard to what it is observing and also make a distinction of time, something the subconscious cannot do. As the patient's conscious mind continues to view the emotional cause of his problem, it begins to understand the connections to his present life. The patient now knows without reservation that this incident occurred a long time ago and should not affect him now, in his present life. Moreover, he realizes it would be foolish for him to continue to suffer as he may have done in that past lifetime.

When the cause of a patient's problem turns out to be a prominent subconscious memory of a highly emotional past life event, the patient's conscious mind may express his understanding in a variety of ways, through statements such as, "So that's it!" or "I'll be damned!"

I once witnessed a highly emotional catharsis by a middle-aged woman who cried incessantly for a full six minutes as her conscious mind integrated what her subconscious had brought up under deep hypnosis. As her tears abated, her face began to take on a radiant glow, and her depressive grimace appeared to transform into a beautiful smile. She then uttered softly, "I'm so relieved! Thank you, thank you," and then shouted, "It's okay to be me!"

THE SUBCONSCIOUS IS INVALUABLE

The more I conduct Comprehensive Hypnoregression Therapy sessions, the more I am convinced that the answers to people's problems lie within the portals of the subconscious mind. Once the subconscious gateway has been entered, I immediately look for a Spirit Guide who is valid and eager to assist me. With such help I am able to identify and interrogate various attached entities and rule in or rule out their very influential involvement in the particular issues that the patient is concerned about. When this has been accomplished and all foreign energy has been properly removed, I then search for an emotional cause of the patient's problems and rely heavily upon the advice of the patient's Spirit Guide.

Looking back, I can honestly say that for a long time I truly believed that for every condition a person has, there is an emotional cause buried deep in the person's subconscious mind, and this held true for both physical and emotional conditions. I held on to this belief as I delved oblivious to the presence and influence of entity attachment. It was not until I discovered that I had regressed an entity attached to the patient, and not the patient, that I took notice that this occurrence required an explanation and a thorough investigation. Since that time I have become very familiar with entity attachments and their releasement and am well aware of their prevalence and of how much they can affect mankind.

The subconscious mind is most assuredly the memory bank that has recorded every moment of every life a person has had; however, my experience with releasement of entities has shown me that it also provides access to one's Higher Self and one's Spirit Guide and any attached entities that happen to be present and affecting that person. I therefore had to modify my statement of belief from, "For every condition a person has, whether it is physical or emotional, there is an emotional cause buried deep in the subconscious mind," to "The cause of physical and emotional conditions that a person may have is buried deep in the subconscious mind." If the person's condition is related to a past memory, it is an emotional cause buried deep in the subconscious. If the person's condition is related to an uninvited entity who is affecting the individual or imprinting its problems upon that person, it is also a cause, and the entity is accessible through the person's subconscious mind. Therefore, the cause may be an emotional memory or an uninvited entity causing the problem, or both.

WHAT MEDICINE NEEDS, AND WHY

Releasing uninvited foreign energy and painful memories can be a monumental step toward curing a person of his emotional or physical ailments and should be an important part of a person's diagnostic investigation. Thus physicians who understand what has been presented here could easily make a referral for a hypnotic subconscious evaluation as commonplace as lab work. By doing so they would be showing the patient that medicine considers the emotional health of the patient to be as important as the health of the patient's body. The therapist who is seeing the patient for this very essential examination should be well trained in what I call Comprehensive Hypnoregression Therapy. All in all, hypnotic past life regression and entity releasement can be an extremely positive, profound, and healing experience, but like everything in medicine, it must be done the right way, which implies that the therapist must not only be well trained but also have knowledge, professionalism, compassion, and a good technique. I predict that the therapists seeing the patients would be comprised of hypnotherapists, retired physicians, physician assistants, and anyone with a passion for truly helping others. Such well-trained individuals would be able to adequately assess a patient's problems and the emotions involved by working with the subconscious mind and making good use of the patient's valid Spirit Guide.

Of great importance is the fact that the therapist needs to know that having a valid Spirit Guide on board is crucial when conducting Comprehensive Hypnoregression Therapy. Following the induction of deep hypnosis, the therapist will then take the patient to his higher self and have him call forth his Spirit Guide and ask for help. If the Spirit Guide comes forth at this time, accepts a gift of Light, and appears to be quite valid, the therapist should first turn his attention to finding out if foreign energy is present, what kind, and how many, and make removal of dark forces an immediate priority. Experience has taught me to deal with the dark forces early because once the dark forces are aware of what's happening, some of them will hide or modify their frequencies to make their discovery by Spirit Guides rather difficult. Once an exorcism of dark force entities has been successfully completed, interrogation of cooperative entities would then be carried out so as to determine if and how much these entities are contributing to the patient's problems. At this point the therapist should look to the Spirit Guide to see if he agrees with the information that has been extracted and if he feels that any of the entities have dark forces attached to them. Uncooperative and hostile entities often do; and if so, a second exorcism is performed. The release of all the remaining entities would follow, using Spirit Guide confirmation for every step of the way, and special techniques for each type of entity, namely seeing that all Earthbound spirits have successfully entered the Light, soul fragments have been sent to their original souls by soul retrieval, and extraterrestrials questioned and convinced to return to their planet with any implants that they have inserted. If extraterrestrials are demonic, they and their implants are removed by exorcism. It is vital that the therapist has Spirit Guide confirmation that all uninvited foreign energy has been sent to their proper destination.

The therapist would then ask the Spirit Guide to check the status of the patient's soul. Is it whole, or has it become fragmented due to trauma in the patient's life? If such fragmentation has occurred in the patient's present life or a past life, a soul retrieval would then be carried out, allowing the patient to once again become a complete soul and thus be less vulnerable to entity infestation. The patient would then be hypnotically instructed to perform a God Light visualization upon waking, before meals, and before going to sleep and an affirmation twice a day and whenever he has a negative thought.

My experience has shown that these protections against future entity attachments really work.

Once the foreign energy problem has been resolved, the therapist would have the patient's Spirit Guide identify the past events that have occurred in the patient's present or past lives that were responsible for, or contributed to, any prominent emotional memory that surfaced and is causing negative programming of the conscious mind. Once the patient is able to review and sometimes relive the emotional moments of his past, his rational conscious mind begins to piece together the connection to his present life, and if such a connection exists, identify relationships that are, in reality, karmic paybacks. The success rate of this therapy will increase and the time utilized during the session will decrease dramatically when a valid Spirit Guide is helping to identify past life occurrences that have contributed to the patient's problems. The therapist must instill within the patient the need for forgiveness of himself and others, and by doing so, help the patient realize that by continuing to wear the heavy chains of unforgiving condemnation he is damaging the health of his mind and his body. The patient must be made to understand that forgiving is not so much for the other person's sake as it is for his own. I have found that forgiveness is extremely powerful and when combined with a very positive attitude it becomes a catalyst for a formula that brings on the law of attraction. Thus more good things will begin to happen in the patient's life and will continue as long as he remains positive and forgiving.

If the prominent emotional memories that surfaced to the forefront of the patient's subconscious mind are not related to karmic issues or important people in the patient's present life, his rational conscious mind makes a distinction of time and understands that these events occurred a long time ago and have no relationship to, or bearing upon, his present life. This knowledge allows the patient's conscious mind to neutralize and therefore delete the negative programming coming from his subconscious mind, thus releasing the effect and the suffering. Revelations such as this are truly life changing.

Powerful suggestions that follow under deep hypnosis enhance the improvement resulting from the release of uninvited entities and painful past memories and if necessary can be used in the future as a reinforcement for all the positive programming that takes place during the session. Finally, protective measures, namely God Light visualization and affirmations are again emphasized in a big way.

If the initial request to have the patient's Spirit Guide come forth is unsuccessful, the therapist should take the patient into a past life and eventually the death experience and once more have the patient call for the Spirit Guide after the patient's soul has entered the Light. I often tell the patient to follow that request with "What is your name, so I may communicate with you?" A few seconds later I then ask the patient what name comes into his mind. This is often successful; however, if it is not, the therapist can call for a volunteer Spirit Guide, possibly Abel, who has come through for me several hundred times. If Abel cannot get through, you can bet the dark forces are the reason, and the patient should be scheduled for a dual hypnosis session.

Patients often feel much lighter and have a greater degree of energy following sessions where their attached entities were released. Patients are often cured following the 2½ to three hour session. If dark forces have interfered to the point of preventing regression and keeping a valid Spirit Guide from coming forth, a dual hypnosis will accomplish what's needed. Thus therapists will need only two sessions at most to help the patient who was referred to them for subconscious evaluation. The patient's subconscious mind will respond in such a positive way that his immune system and autonomic body processes will be energized to the point that the patient will find himself well on the path to physical improvement.

Patients often have a big smile on their face and feel a sense of relief upon waking from their altered state of consciousness. One patient described the experience as a hypnotic adventure into the archives of his subconscious mind. Not only have patients rid themselves of so-called incurable problems that have plagued them for a good part of their life, they have also discovered much about themselves and their loved ones, even those who are deceased. They have experienced lifetimes where they had a talent they were unaware of, lifetimes with loved ones, lifetimes as royalty, in poverty, on other planets; the list is endless.

As a physician, my hope is that people will look upon emotional past memories and possessions by different entities as a disease which can affect our mind, our body, and our personality in a detrimental way. Those that are spiritually enlightened will also realize that entity possessions can affect our souls as well, especially if dark forces are involved. My experience has shown that 70% to 80% of people will have entity attachments at some time in their life. I therefore call upon all physicians to be open minded enough to understand the value of including Comprehensive Hypnoregression in a patient's workup and also understand that this form of investigative and therapeutic use of the subconscious mind will usually bring on great improvement in the patient's condition, often achieving a cure.

Truly, modern conventional medicine needs to make use of the healing power of the patient's subconscious mind as an investigative and diagnostic tool, which can also be therapeutic. Lives would be saved by removing dark forces from suicidal patients, the expense of unnecessary testing would be reduced through early diagnosis, many patients will be cured, and much in the way of suffering would be relieved. This has been my experience.

BIBLIOGRAPHY

Amorth, Fr. Gabriele. *An Exorcist Tells His Story.* Ignatius Press, San Francisco, 1999

Baglio, Matt. *The Rite.* Doubleday, New York, 2009

Baldwin, William. *Healing Lost Souls*, Hampton Roads, Charlottesville, VA. 2003

Baldwin, William. *Spirit Releasement Therapy*, Headline Books, Terra Alta, WV, 1991

Cuneo, St. Michael W. (Jan 1999). "Exorcism." *Contemporary American Religion* 1 (New York: Macmillan Reference USA)

Fiore, Edith. *The Unquiet Dead.* Ballantine: New York, 1995

Leininger, Bruce and Andrea, with Ken Gross. *Soul Survivor.* Grand Central Publishing: New York, 2009

Martin M. *The Roman Ritual of Exorcism.* Harper San Francisco, 1976. Appendix one

Mishlove, Jeffrey. *The Roots of Consciousness: The Classic Encyclopedia of Consciousness Studies Revised and Expanded*, Council Oak Books, OK, 1993

McGill, Ormand. *Hypnotherapy Encyclopedia*, Creativity Unlimited Press, Palos Verdes, CA, 2001

Montgomery, Ruth. *Strangers Among Us.* Fawcett Crest Books, New York, 1979

Montgomery, Ruth, and Joanne Garland. *Ruth Montgomery: Herald of the New Age*, Fawcett Crest Books, New York 1986

Moody, Raymond. *Life After Life*, Bantam Books, New York, 1975

Newton, Michael. *Journey of Souls*, Llewellyn Publications, St. Paul, MN, 2001

Pearsall, Paul. *The Heart's Code*, Random House, New York, 1999

Sutphen, Dick, and Lauren Leigh Taylor. *Past Life Therapy in Action*, Valley of the Sun Publishing Company, Malibu, CA, 1983

Tramont, C. V. *From Birth to ReBirth*, Granite Publishing, Columbus, NC, 2008

Weiss, Brian. *Many Lives, Many Masters*, Simon & Schuster, Inc., New York, 1988 ——*Only Love is Real: A Story of Soulmates Reunited*, Grand Central Publishing, New York, 1997

Woolger, Roger. *Other Lives, Other Selves*, A Dolphin Book: Doubleday, New York, 1987

INDEX

Walk-in phenomenon, 173-174,
    176, 178-180, 184-188, 190
Walk-through phenomenon,
    173-176

Weiss, Brian, 15
World Health Organization, 4

Xenoglossy, 17

ABOUT THE AUTHOR

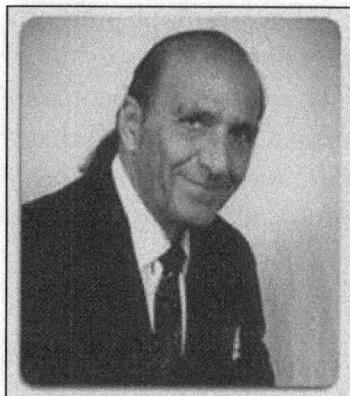

Dr. Tramont received his Bachelor of Science degree from John Carroll University in Cleveland and his M.D. from New York Medical College in New York City. Returning to Cleveland, he completed his internship and a residency in Obstetrics and Gynecology.

After serving two years on active duty deployment in the Air Force during the Vietnam War, he went on to enjoy a fruitful and successful medical practice of 32 years in northeastern Ohio. Positions held during his many years in practice included: President of the County Medical Society, Chief of Obstetrics and Gynecology, Head of the Department of Surgery, and Vice Chief of Staff.

Air Force Reserve accomplishments were inclusive of Fight Surgeon wings following graduation from the School of Aerospace Medicine, graduation from Air War College, appointment to Squadron Commander, promotion to Colonel, and active duty deployment during Desert Storm.

Dr. Tramont has conducted extensive past life research and has carried out past life regression sessions on a part-time basis in conjunction with his medical practice and full-time since he retired to Las Vegas in the year 2000. He is certified by the American Board of Hypnotherapy and has lectured extensively to various groups of people including physicians at Sunrise Hospital in Las Vegas and students at Dr. Raymond Moody's Consciousness Studies classes at the University of Nevada in Las Vegas. Dr. Tramont's first book, *From Birth to ReBirth: Gnostic Healing for the 21st Century*, came out in the year 2009 and has resulted in many radio interviews, including George Noory's Coast to Coast AM.

Dr. Tramont presently carries on an active hypnotherapy practice in Las Vegas using what he calls *Comprehensive Hypnoregression Therapy* to treat people's emotional and physical disorders without drugs. He has found that this form of therapy is able to diagnose and cure most emotional problems and a significant number of physical problems that conventional medicine cannot help.